Textbook for Orthodontic Therapists

Textbook for Orthodontic Therapists

Ceri Davies

Medicine and Dentistry School
University of Central Lancashire
Preston, UK

WILEY Blackwell

This edition first published 2020
© 2020 John Wiley & Sons Ltd

Registered Office(s)
John Wiley & Sons, Inc., 111 River Street, Hoboken, NJ 07030, USA
John Wiley & Sons Ltd, The Atrium, Southern Gate, Chichester, West Sussex, PO19 8SQ, UK

Editorial Office
9600 Garsington Road, Oxford, OX4 2DQ, UK

For details of our global editorial offices, customer services, and more information about Wiley products visit us at www.wiley.com.

Wiley also publishes its books in a variety of electronic formats and by print-on-demand. Some content that appears in standard print versions of this book may not be available in other formats.

Library of Congress Cataloging-in-Publication Data

Names: Davies, Ceri (Orthodontic therapist), author.
Title: Textbook for orthodontic therapists / Ceri Davies.
Description: First edition. | Hoboken, NJ : John Wiley & Sons, 2020. |
   Includes bibliographical references and index.
Identifiers: LCCN 2019045137 (print) | LCCN 2019045138 (ebook) | ISBN
   9781119565451 (paperback) | ISBN 9781119565444 (adobe pdf) | ISBN
   9781119565437 (epub)
Subjects: MESH: Orthodontics–methods | Tooth Diseases–therapy |
   Orthodontic Appliances
Classification: LCC RK521 (print) | LCC RK521 (ebook) | NLM WU 400 | DDC
   617.6/43–dc23
LC record available at https://lccn.loc.gov/2019045137
LC ebook record available at https://lccn.loc.gov/2019045138

Cover Design: Wiley
Cover Images: Dentist examining patiet © Victoria Spendlove, Dental x ray image © Ceri Davies, Teeth bonding © Ceri Davies

Set in 9.5/12.5pt STIXTwoText by SPi Global, Pondicherry, India
Printed and bound in Singapore by Markono Print Media Pte Ltd

10 9 8 7 6 5 4 3 2 1

Contents

Foreword

It was a great honour to have been asked to prepare this foreword for the very first edition of a textbook specifically aimed at orthodontic therapists.

In the past decade, orthodontics as a whole has increased exponentially and hence the demand for orthodontic therapists has proportionally increased. They have to cover a large aspect of orthodontics, similar to a three-year postgraduate orthodontic degree, but in a third the time and almost as much information!

I recommend this book to all orthodontic therapists as it is designed to impart clinical and theoretical knowledge effectively into daily clinical practice. Most importantly it has the best interests of existing and future generations of patients in mind.

The goal of the author has been to put forward information in a logical sequence that will help train both experienced and training therapists alike.

The layout facilitates ease of learning and clinical rationale.

Well done, Ceri!

Dr Shivani Patel
Specialist Orthodontist
BDS(Hons) MFDS RCPS MSc(Lond) IMOrth RCS FDS RCPS FICD(Hons)
London, May 2019

Success doesn't just come and find you, you have to go out and get it

—KUSHANDWIZDOM

Acknowledgements

Firstly, I would like to give a very special thanks to Dr Monica Reinach, who has given me the opportunity to progress my career into becoming an orthodontic therapist. If it was not for Monica I would not be where I am today and I cannot thank her enough for all the support she has given me over the years I worked alongside her at Pure Orthodontics.

Another special thanks goes to Dr Hemant Patel and Chris Cook, my course tutors at university, in helping me to get this book published. All your help and time are very much appreciated. As well, thank you for all your help at university while I was training.

Dr Shivani Patel, your help has been truly appreciated and thank you for helping me in getting this book published.

Thank you to Chris Kimberly from The Specialist Orthodontic Services Lab in Manningtree, Essex, for providing me with some of the photographs used within the Removable Appliance section.

My final thanks go to my work colleagues, who helped me between my clinical sessions in allowing me to use them for some of the photographs in this book. Thank you to every single one of you.

1

History of Orthodontics

The practice of orthodontics, as we know it today, is not just about correcting the position of misaligned teeth, but has a long history behind it. Teeth are important to us, and even in ancient times they were of interest. Archaeologists have found attempts to straighten teeth on human skulls, which had wire wrapped around the teeth in an attempt to realign them. It has taken the knowledge and written works of many dentists and orthodontists to reach the current state of the science.

1.1 Orthodontics before the Twenty-First Century

Modern orthodontics began developing around the eighteenth and nineteenth centuries, but was not known as a specialism until 1900. The appliances that were developed and used over that time were very different to the appliances we use today. A French dentist named Pierre Fauchard designed the first expansion appliance in 1723, which was known as the Bandeau. This consisted of a U-shaped metal strip to which the teeth were ligated. The ligation helped to create expansion. In the late eighteenth century, an American dentist, Norman W. Kingsley, started using an early form of headgear, a traction device to help move teeth distally. The very first type of headgear was created in 1840 and was known as the chin cup. Removable appliances were not used much at this time due to the retention making stability poor. It was not until 1949, when Adams clasps were introduced, that their use became more widespread. A Dwinelle's jack screw was a popular screw to use within removable appliances in the nineteenth century, quite similar to the screws we use on patients today.

Functional appliances only started to be developed in 1879 and again this was by Norman W. Kingsley. The functionals we know today work by posturing the mandible forward, whereas Kingsley designed one that would make the bite jump into the desired position. After this, many more functional appliances were produced, some removable and others fixed. Examples of removable functionals are the monobloc by Pierre Robin in 1902, the medium opening activator by Viggo Andresen in 1990 and the Frankel functional appliances FR-1, FR-2 and FR3, all designed by Rolf Frankel in 1957. An example of a fixed functional is the Herbst, produced in 1905 by Emil Herbst. Clark's twin block is a very popular functional appliance, still used today due to being well tolerated by most patients. This was developed by William Clark and has been used since the 1980s. Fixed appliances were employed very regularly by 1970, although they were slightly different from those we use today.

Edward Angle produced a number of appliances, including in 1904 Angle's E (expansion) arch, which consisted of molar bands with a labial archwire connecting from one molar band to the other running across the labial aspect of the dentition. Teeth needing expansion were then ligated to the archwire. Around 1910 Angle realised that he needed more control of the teeth, so to gain this he developed the pin and tube appliance. Gold and platinum bands were used on all the teeth with a vertical tube soldered onto them, then a pin was used which passed through this tube, achieving tooth movement. The downside of this was that rotational movement and root parallelism were difficult to achieve due to the use of round archwires. The pins had to be removed and resoldered into a new position at every appointment. The ribbon arch was the next appliance that Angle developed in 1915. With this rotational movement was achievable due to the vertical bracket soldered onto each band. Raymond Begg was inspired by this appliance and went on to develop his lightwire technique from it. Five years before Angle died in 1930, his final invention was the edgewise appliance, which was a bracket with a horizontal slot that was identical for every tooth. Angle moved away from the vertical slot, since he found that using a horizontal slot meant rectangular archwires could be used and by placing bends this allowed three-dimensional control of the teeth. The preadjusted edgewise appliance used today is based on Angle's edgewise appliance.

During the twentieth century fixed appliances consisted of bands with brackets welded onto them. Bands were made chairside by using straight strips of stainless steel that were shaped for each individual tooth, but as you might imagine this was very time consuming. In 1930 these stainless steel bands began being sold ready made by the very first orthodontic supply company. The purpose of the bracket was to hold the archwire in place. Tooth movement was achieved by the orthodontist placing bends within the archwire. Again, this was very time consuming and it took hours to get fixed appliances onto a patient.

In 1970, Lawrence Andrews developed the preadjusted edgewise appliance which is still popular today, and this changed much in orthodontics. The difference with this appliance was that the brackets were made for each specific tooth and contained prescriptions such as in and out, tip and torque within the bracket. These prescriptions all helped with tooth movement and reduced the need for wire bending. Today these prescription brackets are available with different angulations, slot sizes and base types.

Aesthetic brackets first become available in 1963, which are very popular today, as are lingual appliances, the first of which were developed in the 1980s. Since then a wide range of different systems have been developed by orthodontists, including the standard edgewise appliance, Begg appliance, tip edge appliance, preadjusted edgewise appliance, self-ligating appliance, and the lingual appliance system. We will look at each of these in turn.

1.2 Standard Edgewise Appliance

Edward Angle (1855–1930):

- Developed the standard edgewise appliance in 1925.
- Was an American dentist and was known as the 'Father of orthodontics'.
- Attended Pennsylvania College of Dental Surgery and qualified in 1878 as a dentist.
- Founded the Angle School of Orthodontia in 1890, where orthodontics become known as a specialism.
- Angle's classification of malocclusion that we use today was developed by him in 1890.
- Established many appliances within his lifetime, such as the E arch appliance (1907), the pin and tube appliance (1910), the ribbon arch appliance (1915) and the edgewise appliance (1925).
- In 1930 he died at the age of 75.

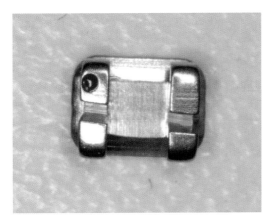

Figure 1.1 Standard edgewise bracket. The same bracket is used for every tooth which contains a passive bracket slot with no inbuilt prescription.

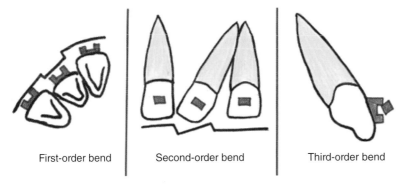

First-order bend   Second-order bend   Third-order bend

Figure 1.2 First-, second-, and third-order bends.

Standard edgewise appliance (Figure 1.1):

- The design of the bracket was the same for every tooth which had a passive bracket slot.
- All brackets were rectangular in shape.
- The size of the bracket was determined by the width of the bracket slot.
- The brackets came in two different sizes:
  – Width usually 0.018 or 0.022 in.
  – Depth usually 0.025 or 0.028 in.
- The appliance had three-dimensional control of the teeth.
- To aid tooth movement all archwires were dependent on bends being added. However, this was time consuming and difficult for the orthodontist, as it was required at every visit.
- The bends created were to achieve the following (Figure 1.2):
  – *First-order bend – in and out:*
    o To compensate for the different tooth widths, bends are placed in the horizontal plane of the archwire.
    o The bends correct the tooth widths in the bucco-lingual and labial-palatal direction (anterio-posterior [AP] plane – anterior/posterior movement, front to back).
    o For example: in modern-day orthodontics, central incisors are always slightly in front of the lateral incisors, which sit slightly back. Canines sit in the same anterio-posterior position as the central incisors, which helps to create the canine eminence (corner of the mouth).

 – *Second-order bend – tip:*
  o To compensate and correct the angulation of the teeth, bends are placed in the vertical plane to achieve the correct mesiodistal angulation of the teeth.
  o For example: distally angulated laterals would need bends to help upright the laterals mesially, which ensures that teeth gain the desired angulation.
 – *Third-order bend – torque (rectangular wire only):*
  o This is achieved with rectangular archwires only.
  o Orthodontists would place a bend in the archwire to help correct the torque of the roots.
  o For example: buccal root torque is achieved by the archwire being twisted forwards; palatal root torque is achieved by the archwire being twisted backwards.
- Closing loops were placed within the archwire and used as a method of space closure.
- This system placed a high demand on anchorage.
  Tooth movement can be effected due to the inter-bracket span, the distance between the brackets:
 – Narrow brackets (more span): a greater span of the archwire between the brackets has the ability to make the archwire more flexible, which can achieve faster alignment.
 – Wider brackets (less span): a reduced span of the archwire between the brackets is more efficient for de-rotation and mesiodistal control of teeth.

1.3 Begg Appliance

P. Raymond Begg (1898–1983):

- Developed the Begg appliance in the 1950s.
- An Australian dentist.
- Attended the Angle School of Orthodontia in Pasadena, California in 1924 and was one of the first at the school to treat patients with the standard edgewise appliance.
- In 1925 he travelled back to Adelaide, South Australia to treat his own patients in orthodontics.
- Became a professor at the University of Adelaide.
- Was also known to develop the Australian orthodontic wires.
- In 1980 he retired and then died in 1983.

Begg appliance (Figure 1.3):

- This appliance was designed to overcome the high anchorage demand of the standard edgewise appliance and is a light anchorage appliance.
- Another name for the Begg appliance is the lightwire appliance.
- The components of the appliance are the bracket, pin, and archwire.

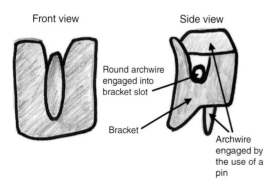

Front view   Side view

Round archwire engaged into bracket slot

Bracket

Archwire engaged by the use of a pin

Figure 1.3 A Begg appliance. The components of the bracket are labelled.

(a)

(b)

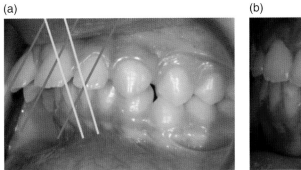
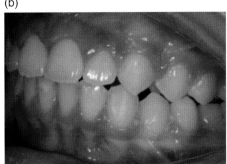

Figure 1.4 How the Begg appliance works. (a) The teeth are tipped into the desired position by the use of inter-maxillary elastics. The lines on the photograph show the inclination of how the upper and lower teeth sit. (b) The roots of these teeth are uprighted by the use of auxiliary springs.

- To ensure full engagement of the archwire, the pin is used to hold the archwire within the bracket slot.
- The appliance is dependent on round archwires only, which fit loosely into the bracket slot at the top of the bracket – this allows a lot of slop (play) within the bracket.
- Final detailing of teeth is difficult to achieve in this type of appliance.

The Begg appliance uses different methods to gain tooth movement (Figure 1.4):

- Round archwires and inter-maxillary elastics tip the teeth into the desired position.
- Auxiliary springs or loops are placed within the archwire to help upright the roots of the teeth and achieve rotational movement.
- To provide intra-oral anchorage, extractions can be considered, since intra-oral elastic wear would use the posterior segment as an anchor unit to help retract the anterior segment.
- Patient compliance is important throughout treatment with this appliance, as it is very dependent on intra-oral elastics.

1.4 Preadjusted Edgewise Appliance

Lawrence Andrews:

- Developed the preadjusted edgewise appliance in 1970.
- Also developed Andrews' six keys to occlusion.
- Is an American orthodontist who has now retired from patient care, although he still takes part in research and education.
- His son Will A. Andrews followed in his footsteps and joined the practice that Lawrence established in 1958 called Point Loma in San Diego, California.

Preadjusted edgewise appliance (Figure 1.5):

- Another name for this is the straight-wire appliance.
- It is used on patients for either their first stage of treatment or the second stage following removable or functional appliances.
- These brackets are called 'preadjusted' edgewise brackets because they are thicker in the horizontal dimension, and are also different from one another due to the inbuilt prescriptions designed specifically for each individual tooth.

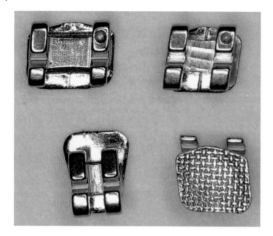

Figure 1.5 Preadjusted edgewise brackets.

- The inbuilt prescriptions within the brackets are:
  - *In and out*: first-order bend
  - *Tip*: second-order bend
  - *Torque*: third-order bend.
- Because of the inbuilt prescriptions within the brackets they became very popular, as it meant wire bending was minimised and in some cases not needed at all.
- For the inbuilt prescriptions to be achieved on each tooth, the brackets are manufactured in a certain way:
  - *In and out (first-order bend)*: to achieve this, the base of the bracket is manufactured differently. For example, lateral incisors sit slightly back from the central incisors, therefore the base of this bracket will be thicker than the brackets for the central incisors.
  - *Tip (second-order bend)*: each bracket slot is cut at a certain angulation to help achieve the correct angulation for each individual tooth; this differs for each bracket.
  - *Torque (third-order bend)*: each bracket has different torque percentages within the bracket slot. The thicker the wire, the more torque is created. If the desired torque is not achieved, bends within archwires can be placed to help with this type of movement.
- Preformed archwires are used with this appliance, as this allows teeth to move gradually from their original position into their desired position.
- Brackets come in different slot sizes:
  - 0.018×0.025 in., with the working wire being used $= 16 \times 22$ ss (stainless steel)
  - 0.022×0.028 in., with the working wire being used $= 19 \times 25$ ss (more commonly used).
- Depending on the degree of crowding the patient presents with, the appliance can be used on non-extraction or extraction cases.
- Still in good use today, the preadjusted edgewise appliance has three common bracket prescriptions:
  - Andrews
  - Roth
  - MBT = McLaughlin, Bennett, Trevisi.
- Different orthodontists created these three common bracket prescriptions. It was known that each orthodontist had different views on how much torque should be built within the bracket slot. Therefore, each bracket prescription contains different values of torque, with MBT containing the highest value of torque out of the three.

Advantages of the edgewise appliance:

- Reduced chair time.
- Amount of wire bending is minimised.
- Sliding mechanics for tooth movement.
- Good finishing.

Disadvantages:

- Larger inventory of brackets is required, as each individual tooth has different requirements of in and out, tip and torque.
- Ignores individual biological variation.
- Increased friction has implications and increases anchorage considerations.

1.5 Tip Edge Appliance

Peter Kelsing:

- Developed the tip edge appliance in 1986.
- Is an American orthodontist, born in La Porte, Indiana, and is the son of Harold Kesling who was also an orthodontist.
- Peter also has one son called Chris Kesling who followed in both his father's and grandfather's footsteps and works as an orthodontist at the same practice in Westville, Indiana.

Tip edge appliance:

- Developed based on the best features of the Begg appliance (round wires, light forces) and the preadjusted edgewise appliance (detailed finishing).
- There are three stages of treatment when using this appliance:
  - *Stage 1*: Align teeth, correct incisor and molar relationship, crossbites and rotations.
  - *Stage 2*: Start space closure and maintain stage 1 corrections.
  - *Stage 3*: Correct inclination of teeth.
- Each bracket incorporates the inbuilt prescriptions (in and out, tip, torque).
- Round archwires are used for the initial tipping and aligning stage and the later stages have the use of the rectangular archwires, which gives more control over tooth movement and helps with the final detailing.
- To ensure full engagement, the archwire is engaged into the bracket slot by the use of elastomeric modules or metal ligatures.

1.6 Self-ligating Appliance

Self-ligating appliance (Figure 1.6):

- Developed in 1990.
- Became very popular among non-extraction orthodontists and was initially used on non-extraction cases.
- Self-ligating brackets incorporate a door/clip which ensures full engagement, and holds the archwire in place within the bracket slot.

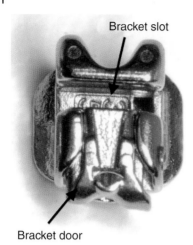

Bracket slot

Bracket door

Figure 1.6   Self-ligating appliance.

- There are two types of self-ligating bracket:
  - *Passive*: has a slide mechanism which is passive and places no active force on the archwire.
  - *Active*: Places an active force on the archwire.
- Once engagement of the archwire has been made by the door/clip, the archwire is free to move in brackets, making the appliance free-sliding.
- The circumference of the arch is increased, due to space being created on expansion to align teeth, leading to the wide smiles we see today.
- Inter-arch elastics are used in conjunction with self-ligating appliances to help improve the patient's occlusion.
- Self-ligating appliances are known to reduce chairside time as adjustments are quicker.
- Different types of torque are available within the brackets, such as standard/high/low torque.
- Manufacturers claim that self-ligating appliances produce lower friction.

Examples of self-ligating systems:

- Damon® – 3, 3mx, Q, Clear (Ormco Corporation, Orange, CA, USA).
- Clarity™ SL (3M, St Paul, MN, USA).
- Harmony (ASO International, Tokyo, Japan).
- SmartClip™ (3M).
- SPEED System™ (Haspeler Orthodontics, Cambridge, ON, Canada).
- In-Ovation C® (Dentsply Sirona, Woodbridge, ON, Canada).

Advantages:

- Provides low friction.
- Achieves full archwire engagement.
- Quick and easy to use.
- No elastomeric modules, which makes oral hygiene easier to control.
- Patient can go for longer intervals between appointments.

Disadvantages:

- If there is a fault in the door/clip, it means the whole bracket is faulty, therefore a new bracket would be needed.
- Appliance can be harder to ligate wire; it is important to make sure the wire is fully engaged in the bracket slot for the door to close.
- Higher cost in brackets.
- Difficulty in finishing due to the incomplete expression of the archwires.

1.7   Advantages and Disadvantages of all Types of Buccal Appliances

Advantages:

- Appliances allow good working access.
- Once the clinician is experienced they are easy to work on.
- Chairside working time is reduced.

- Can achieve excellent finishing and detailing – archwire bending is easier.
- Aesthetic brackets and archwires, which are popular with patients.
- Quicker treatment time as opposed to lingual appliances.

Disadvantages:

- Poor aesthetics as they are on the labial/buccal surface of teeth.
- Any decalcification occurring from treatment will be visible.
- Aesthetic brackets can fracture during debonding.

1.8 Lingual Appliances

Lingual appliances (Figure 1.7):

- First developed in the 1970s in the USA.
- The brackets are bonded onto the palatal/lingual surface of the upper and lower arches.
- Lingual appliances use preadjusted ribbonwise brackets, which are thicker vertically than horizontally.
- All brackets and archwires are custom made to reduce speech problems and tongue irritation and to help improve finishing.
- Custom-made brackets are good as they can be rebonded directly back on if they debond during treatment; however, if a bracket is lost, new ones have to be specially ordered.
- Brackets come in a jig and are all bonded together at once (indirect bonding). It is important to keep the bracket in the jig, because there can be undesired tooth movement if it comes out or is bonded directly to the tooth without a jig.
- Lingual appliances can also come in a self-ligating form.

Advantages:

- Good aesthetics.
- Decalcification less likely to occur with lingual appliances compared to labial appliances; however, if present it will not be visible.
- Upper anterior brackets can act as a bite plane, which is good for treating overbites (flat anterior bite plane or FABP).

Disadvantages:

- Can affect patient's speech.
- Much more ulceration can appear.
- Discomfort to patient's tongue.
- Clinically demanding on clinicians.
- Inter-bracket span is reduced.
- Increased chairside time.
- Finishing and detailing are difficult to achieve due to the reduced inter-bracket span, and archwire bending can be made difficult.
- Indirect bonding of brackets or debonding of brackets can result in poor positioning if not bonded back in the correct position.
- Increased cost.
- Longer treatment time.

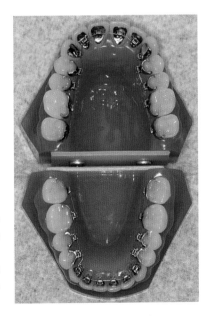

Figure 1.7 Typhodont showing Harmony lingual appliance.

2

Patient Assessment

Patient assessment is very important prior to orthodontic treatment. Including radiographs and study models, each patient should have an orthodontic assessment. This assessment looks at the patient's skeletal features and malocclusion. Assessment must be done to help the orthodontist assess the need for treatment and create a treatment plan that is appropriate to the patient.

A patient assessment is done in two ways:

- Extra-oral assessment
- Intra-oral assessment.

The three planes of space are used when carrying out the assessments. The extra-oral assessment refers to outside the mouth, whereas the intra-oral looks inside the mouth. The two assessments consider the following:

- *Extra-oral assessment*: assesses the facial profile.
- *Intra-oral assessment*: assesses the position of the upper and lower dentition.

2.1 The Three Planes of Space

The three planes of space we refer to in orthodontics are:

- *Antero-posterior plane* (AP): assesses the patient front to back.
- *Vertical plane*: assesses the patient up and down.
- *Transverse (horizontal) plane*: assesses the patient side to side.

2.2 Extra-Oral Assessment

There are four stages to carrying out an extra-oral assessment. The first three look at the three planes of space, whereas the fourth stage concentrates on the lower third of the face.

Textbook for Orthodontic Therapists, First Edition. Ceri Davies.
© 2020 John Wiley & Sons Ltd. Published 2020 by John Wiley & Sons Ltd.

2.2.1 Antero-posterior Plane

- The patient is viewed from the side.
- This stage looks at the patient's skeletal pattern in the AP plane (front to back).
- It assesses the patient's profile and the relationship of the maxilla, referred to as the A point, and the mandible, referred to as the B point.
-

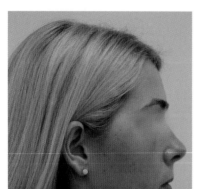

Patients are assessed by the following:
- *Skeletal class I*: Mandible is 2–3 mm posterior to the maxilla (Figure 2.1).
- *Skeletal class II*: Mandible is retruded relative to the maxilla (Figure 2.2).
- *Skeletal class III*: Mandible is protruded relative to the maxilla (Figure 2.3).

2.2.2 Vertical Plane

- The patient is viewed from the front and side.
- This stage looks at the patient's skeletal pattern in the vertical plane (up and down).
- It assesses the lower part of the face, looking at the LAFH (lower anterior facial height) and FMPA (Frankfort-mandibular plane angle).

LAFH:
- LAFH should measure the same as UAFH (upper anterior facial height).

Figure 2.1 Skeletal class I.

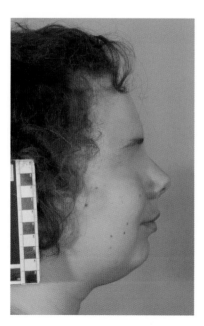

Figure 2.2 Skeletal class II.

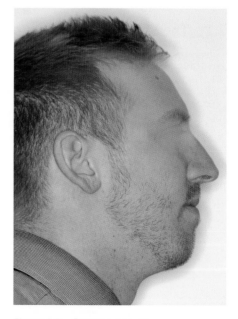

Figure 2.3 Skeletal class III.

- UAFH is measured from the eyebrow to the base of nose (Figure 2.4).
- LAFH is measured from the base of the nose to the lowest point on the chin.

FMPA:

- This is the angle where the Frankfort plane and mandibular plane meet (Figure 2.5).
- This is assessed by placing one hand on the Frankfort plane and one hand on the mandibular plane and assessing where they cross by eye.

  The measurements indicate the following:
  - Average LAFH and FMPA – usually seen in class I.
  - Decreased LAFH and low FMPA – usually seen in class II.
  - Increased LAFH and high FMPA – usually seen in class III.

2.2.3 Transverse Plane

- The patient is viewed from the front and looking down on the face from above.
- This stage looks at the patient's skeletal pattern in the transverse plane (side to side).
- This is assessed by looking at the patient's face and recording any significant asymmetry (Figure 2.6) – all patients are asymmetrical.

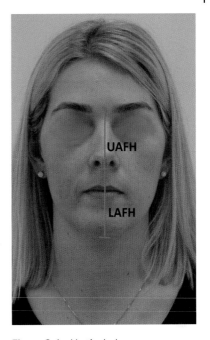

Figure 2.4 Vertical plane measurements: frontal view.

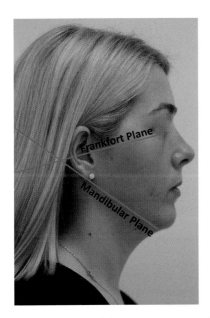

Figure 2.5 Vertical plane measurements: right profile.

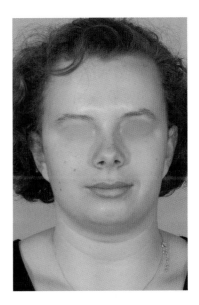

Figure 2.6 Transverse plane: frontal view looking for any asymmetry.

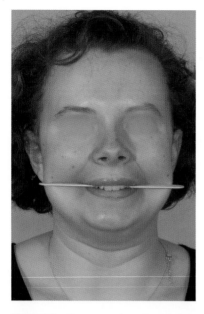

Figure 2.7 Transverse plane: frontal view looking for any asymmetry with a spatula.

- To assess whether the occlusal plane follows the line of asymmetry, a tongue spatula is used and the patient is asked to bite onto this (Figure 2.7). In patients who have a significant asymmetry, this will be noticeable by the tongue spatula not lying flat.

2.2.4 Profile Pattern

- This is assessed by looking at the LAFH.
- Patients can present with different profiles: concave, straight, or convex (Figure 2.8).
- In the convex profile the LAFH is protruded, most commonly found in African Caribbean people.
- In the straight profile the LAFH is straight from the nose to the chin.
- In the concave profile the LAFH is caved in between the nose and the chin.
- Patients with a concave profile should be approached with care when it comes to extractions, as this could make them even more concave, whereas convex profile patients would benefit from this.

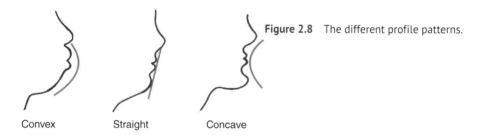

Convex   Straight   Concave

Figure 2.8 The different profile patterns.

2.3 Intra-Oral Assessment

There are many stages considered when carrying out an intra-oral assessment. The first three look at the three planes of space, whereas the remaining eight look more into how the dentition appears in the mouth.

2.3.1 Anterio-posterior Plane

- Assesses the arch from front to back.
- This stage looks at the different types of relationships of the occlusion, such as molar relationship, incisor relationship, canine relationship, and overjet.
- Molar relationship:
  - Also known as Angle's classification.
  - Looks at the position of the upper first molars.
  - Classification is class I; class II, II25, II50, II70; and class III, III25, III50, III70.

- Incisor relationship:
  - Also known as the BSIC (British Standards Institute Classification 1983).
  - Looks at the position of the incisors.
  - Classification is Class I; Class II div I, div II; and Class III.
- Canine relationship:
  - Looks at the position of the canines.
  - Classification is class I; class II, II25 II50, II70; and class III, III25, III50, III70.
- Overjet:
  - Distance between the upper and lower teeth within the horizontal plane. The distance between them is measured with a stainless-steel ruler.

2.3.2   Vertical Plane

- Assesses the arch up and down.
- Looks at the overbite.
- The overbite is the vertical overlap of the upper incisors over the lower incisors when the posterior teeth are in occlusion. It can be measured as:
  - *Average*: upper incisors cover one-third of the lower incisors when in occlusion.
  - *Increased and complete*: upper incisors cover more than one-third of the lower incisors, but are complete (touching) on hard or soft tissues when in occlusion.
  - *Increased and incomplete*: upper incisors cover more than one-third of the lower incisors and are incomplete (not touching) on hard or soft tissues when in occlusion.
  - *Decreased and complete*: upper incisors cover less than one-third of the lower incisors, but are complete (touching) on hard or soft tissues when in occlusion.
  - *Decreased and incomplete*: upper incisors cover less than one-third of the lower incisors and are incomplete (not touching) on hard or soft tissues when in occlusion.

2.3.3   Transverse Plane

- Assesses the arch from side to side.
- Looks for any posterior crossbites.
- A posterior crossbite is found when the upper dentition on the posterior segment sits within the lower teeth when occluding.
- There can be unilateral or bilateral crossbites, unilateral meaning on one side of the arch and bilateral being on both sides of the arch.

2.3.4   Crowding

- This assesses the amount of crowding there is within both the upper and lower arches.
- Assessing the crowding falls into the category of space analysis.
- Constructing an archform that best fits the majority of the teeth can help analyse how much crowding there is within the arch.
- Once the archform has been constructed, it is then measured by the use of floss and a stainless-steel ruler. Once the measurement has been calculated for that, the mesiodistal widths of all the teeth within that arch are measured. The calculations are then taken away from each other, which gives you the total amount of crowding:

    Mesiodistal widths − constructed archform = total crowding

- Crowding is then classified as the following:
  - *Mild crowding*: 2–4 mm
  - *Moderate crowding*: 4–8 mm
  - *Severe crowding*: 8+ mm.

2.3.5 Spacing

- This assesses the amount of spacing that is present within the two arches.
- Spacing can be classified into mild, moderate, or severe.
  Spacing can be found within the arch due to the following:
  - *Extractions*: patients who have previously had extractions, for example extracted LL6.
  - *Dento-alveolar disproportion*: patients who have big arches but small (microdontia) teeth can present with spacing between the teeth.
  - *Microdontia*: patient who present with small teeth, for example peg laterals.
  - *Diastema*: patients who present with a diastema within the arch, which could be due to a habit such as thumb sucking, active tongue thrust, or a mesiodens lying erupted or unerupted between the upper central incisors.

2.3.6 Path of Closure

- This assesses how the patient bites the teeth together.
- When assessing the bite we look at:
  - Is there any deviation of the mandible on closing?
  - Does it shift left, right, or forward to gain a comfortable bite?

2.3.7 Teeth Present/Missing

- This will look at how many teeth there are.
- Patients can present with missing teeth or extra teeth.
- Missing teeth could be for numerous reasons:
  - Hypodontia cases
  - Previous extractions
  - Impacted teeth.
- Extra teeth could be due to supernumerary teeth such as:
  - Conical teeth, also known as mesiodens
  - Tuberculates
  - Supplemental teeth
  - Odontomes.

2.3.8 Habits

- This stages assesses if the patient has any habits that may affect the teeth, such as thumb sucking or a tongue thrust.
- It is important to establish whether the patient has a relevant habit or not prior to treatment starting.
- All habits must be ceased before orthodontic treatment can be commenced, as continuing could increase the length of treatment and, more importantly, result in relapse at the end of treatment.

2.3.9   PPP – Presence, Position, Pathology

- *Presence* looks at what teeth are present in the mouth.
- *Position* looks at the position of the teeth, such as impacted teeth, rotated teeth, or palatally/buccally displaced teeth.
- *Pathology* looks at the health of the teeth, for instance any caries that could be present which would necessitate fillings. This area can also highlight any dental health problems, for example any recession, erosion, gum disease, or even gingivitis that a patient may have; it is important to identify this prior to treatment to make sure it is fully under control. Any more underlying problems found around the apical area of a tooth can be identified by the use of appropriate radiographs.

2.3.10   SSC – Size, Shape, Colour

- This stage looks at the size, shape, and colour of all teeth, for example:
  - Microdontia: small teeth
  - Macrodontia: big teeth
  - Peg laterals
  - Trauma to teeth resulting in nerve death and causing discoloration of the teeth.

2.3.11   Temporal Mandibular Joint

- This stage assesses the jaw.
- Does the patient have any problems with the temporal mandibular joint on opening and closing?
- Has the patient reported any symptoms?
- Do they experience any clicking or pain?

3

Classification of Malocclusion

Classification of malocclusion looks at the position of the teeth when the patient is in occlusion. These classifications look at the relationship of how the molars, incisors, and canines meet.

They are categorized into three groups:

- Angle's classification
- British Standards Institute classification
- Canine relationship.

3.1   Angle's Classification

Developed by Edward Angle in 1899, this type of classification looks at the antero-posterior position of the first permanent molars, known as the molar relationship.

- *Class I*: the mesiobuccal cusp of the upper first molar occludes in the buccal groove of the lower first molar (Figure 3.1).
- *Class II*: the mesiobuccal cusp of the upper first molar occludes anterior to the buccal groove of the lower first molar (Figure 3.2).
- *Class III*: the mesiobuccal cusp of the upper first molar occludes posterior to the buccal groove of the lower first molar (Figure 3.3).
- *Class II25*: the mesiobuccal cusp of the upper first molar occludes one-quarter anterior to the buccal groove of the lower first molar.
- *Class II50*: the mesiobuccal cusp of the upper first molar occludes half a unit anterior to the buccal groove of the lower first molar (cusp to cusp with the lower first molar).
- *Class II75*: the mesiobuccal cusp of the upper first molar occludes three-quarters anterior to the buccal groove of the lower first molar (not a full unit class II).
- *Class III25*: the mesiobuccal cusp of the upper first molar occludes one-quarter posterior to the buccal groove of the lower first molar.
- *Class III50*: the mesiobuccal cusp of the upper first molar occludes half a unit posterior to the buccal groove of the lower first molar (cusp to cusp with the lower second molar).
- *Class III75*: the mesiobuccal cusp of the upper first molar occludes three-quarters posterior to the buccal groove of the lower first molar (not a full unit class III).

Textbook for Orthodontic Therapists, First Edition. Ceri Davies.
© 2020 John Wiley & Sons Ltd. Published 2020 by John Wiley & Sons Ltd.

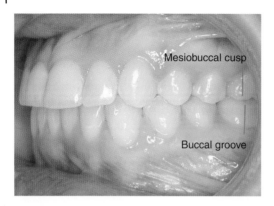

Figure 3.1 Class I molar relationship.

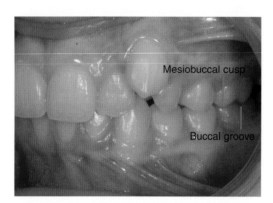

Figure 3.2 Class II molar relationship.

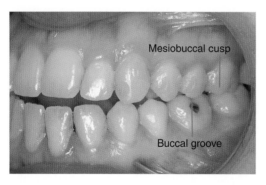

Figure 3.3 Class III molar relationship.

3.2 British Standards Institute Classification

This type of classification looks at the incisor relationship.

- *Class I*: the lower incisor edges occlude with or lie immediately below the cingulum plateau of the upper central incisors (Figure 3.4).

- *Class II div I*: the lower incisor edges occlude posterior to the cingulum plateau of the upper central incisors. The upper central incisors are proclined and there is an increase in the overjet (Figure 3.5).
- *Class II div II*: the lower incisors edges occlude posterior to the cingulum plateau of the upper central incisors. The upper central incisors are retroclined and there is a reduced or increased overjet (Figure 3.6). A common feature is proclined lateral incisors.
- *Class III*: the lower incisor edges occlude anterior to the cingulum plateau of the upper central incisors. The overjet is reduced or reversed (Figure 3.7).

3.3 Canine Relationship

This classification looks at the position of the canine.

- *Class I*: the upper canine occludes and lies in the embrasure between the lower canine and first premolar (Figure 3.8).
- *Class II*: the upper canine occludes anteriorly and lies in the embrasure between the lower lateral incisors and the canine (Figure 3.9).
- *Class III*: the upper canine occludes posteriorly and lies in the embrasure between the lower first and second premolars (Figure 3.10).
- *Class II25*: the upper canine occludes one-quarter anteriorly from being in embrasure between the lower lateral incisors and the canine.
- *Class II50*: the upper canine occludes half a unit anteriorly and lies directly over the lower canine (cusp to cusp with the lower canine).
- *Class II75*: the upper canine occludes three-quarters anteriorly from being in embrasure between the lower lateral incisors and the canine (not a full unit class II).
- *Class III25*: the upper canine occludes one-quarter posteriorly from being in embrasure between the lower first and second premolars.
- *Class III50*: the upper canine occludes half a unit posteriorly and lies directly between the lower first and second premolars.
- *Class III75*: the upper canine occludes three-quarters posteriorly from being in embrasure between the lower first and second premolars (not a full unit class III).

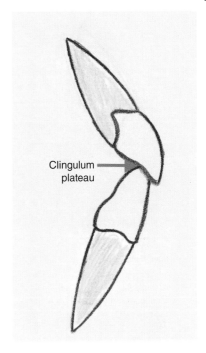

Clingulum plateau

Figure 3.4 Incisor relationship class I.

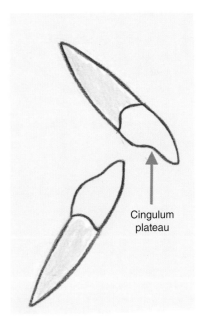

Cingulum plateau

Figure 3.5 Incisor relationship class II div I.

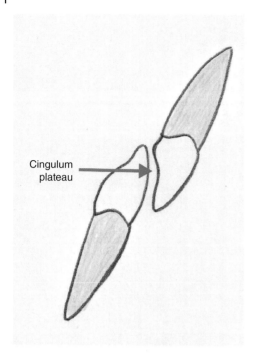

Figure 3.6   Incisor relationship class II div II.

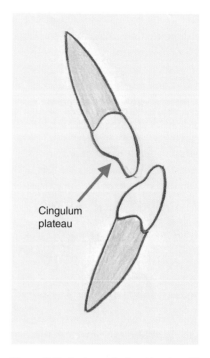

Figure 3.7   Incisor relationship class III.

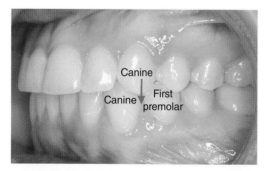

Figure 3.8   Class I canine relationship.

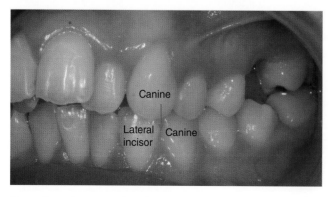

Figure 3.9   Class II canine relationship.

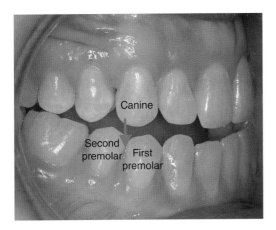

Figure 3.10   Class III canine relationship.

3.4   Andrew's Six Keys

This classification was developed by Lawrence Andrews, the same orthodontist who developed the preadjusted edgewise appliance. Over time Andrews decided that it was not always possible to achieve a good class I occlusion, therefore the six keys were developed to identify each feature to evaluate why this was not possible. A seventh key was added subsequently because correct tooth size can have an effect on achieving good class I occlusion.

1) Correct molar relationship:
   - The mesiobuccal cusp of the upper first molar occludes in the buccal groove of the lower first molar.
   - The distobuccal cusp of the upper first molar occludes on the mesiobuccal cusp of the lower second molar.
2) Correct crown angulation:
   - All tooth crowns are angulated mesially.
3) Correct crown inclination:
   - Incisors are inclined towards the buccal or labial surface.
   - Buccal segment teeth are inclined lingually; in the lower buccal segments this is progressive.
4) Flat curve of Spee.
5) No rotations.
6) No spaces.
7) Correct tooth size.

4

Aetiology of Malocclusion

This chapter will look at all the different types of causes for the types of malocclusions we see in orthodontics.

4.1 Skeletal Factors

Skeletal factors are categorised into all three planes of space.

4.1.1 Anteroposterior Plane (AP)

Dento-alveolar compensation is a term used when teeth compensate for the skeletal pattern. For example, a patient may have class I incisors but be presenting with a class III skeletal pattern.

4.1.2 Vertical Plane

Growth rotations occur in the mandible. This is extra growth which can be seen once the patient has stopped growing. There are two types:

- Forward growth rotation – decreased lower anterior facial height (LAFH).
- Backward growth rotation – increased LAFH.

4.1.3 Transverse Plane

Absolute transverse maxillary deficiency:

- This term relates to crossbites and is most commonly seen in class III cases.
- Commonly seen in maxillary retrusion, this is where the maxilla is reduced in all three dimensions, which can result in crossbites anteriorly and posteriorly.

Dento-alveolar compensation:

- This term is used when teeth compensate for the skeletal pattern.
- In this case transversely, teeth can compensate to result in a crossbite being present.
- For example, tipping of the buccal surface of the upper molar and lingual surface of the lower molar compensates for transverse maxillary deficiency.

Textbook for Orthodontic Therapists, First Edition. Ceri Davies.
© 2020 John Wiley & Sons Ltd. Published 2020 by John Wiley & Sons Ltd.

4.2 Soft Tissue Factors

4.2.1 Fullness and Tone of the Lips

The fullness and tone of lips can have an effect on the dentition, as they can result in positioning of the incisors in the labiolingual direction. The effects can include the following:

- Lips that lack muscular tone and are flaccid – incisors tend to be proclined.
- Strap-like lips:
  - Lips are tense and the incisors tend to be retroclined.
  - The term highly active lip can also be used to describe this.
- Lower lip line:
  - The lower lip should cover one-third to one-half of the upper incisor crowns.
  - More than one-half coverage = retroclined upper incisors.
  - Less than one-third coverage = proclined upper incisors.

4.2.2 Lip Competency

Lip competency looks at how the lips are when the patient is at rest. There are two types of lip competency:

- Competent lips, which is where minimal effort is required to achieve an oral seal.
- Incompetent lips, which is where excessive muscular activity is required to achieve an oral seal.
- With incompetent lips the following features can be found:
  - Can often be associated with a low lower lip line.
  - Swallowing patterns may occur to achieve an anterior oral seal. If excessive muscular activity or forward mandibular posturing is not possible to achieve, then the following swallowing patterns can occur:
    o Tongue to lower lip results in incisor proclination.
    o Lower lip to palate results in upper incisor proclination and lower incisor retroclination.
    o Tongue to upper lip results in upper incisor proclination.

4.2.3 Macroglossia (Large Tongue)

The size of the tongue can affect the development of the dentition. The tongue can also impede incisor eruption and anterior open bite (AOB). The tongue can present with two types of tongue thrusts:

- Adaptive tongue thrust: this can be corrected and stopped once the positions of the teeth are corrected. It is seen when the tongue is forced between the teeth.
- Endogenous tongue thrust: this is where the tongue is thrusted forward between the teeth, but is a habit that may not be stopped once tooth positions have been corrected. This can result in relapse.

4.2.4 Enlarged Adenoids

Adenoids are large glands which are located by the soft palate in the roof of the mouth. Enlarged adenoids can result in the development of an AOB due to constant mouth breathing. This has the effect of the molars over-erupting and resulting in an increased LAFH.

4.2.5 Generalised Pathology of Muscles

Muscle weakness can also have an effect on the dentition. Weak muscles enable the teeth to move due to the lack of support of the soft tissues surrounding the dentition.

4.3 Local Factors

Local factors are divided into three groups:

- Variation in tooth number
- Variation in tooth size
- Variation in tooth position.

4.3.1 Variation in Tooth Number

4.3.1.1 Hypodontia

- Hypodontia is known as missing teeth.
- Hypodontia is found when there is an absence of one or more primary or secondary teeth, excluding third molars.
- The most common cause can be genetic, with a family history of hypodontia.
- The most common missing teeth are upper third molars (U8s), lower third molars (L8s), lower premolars (L5s), upper lateral incisors (U2s), upper premolars (U5s), and lower central incisors (L1s).

4.3.1.2 Supernumerary

- Supernumerary teeth are extra teeth.
- Supernumerary teeth are found when there are excessive teeth in the normal series.
- The most commonly found supernumerary is in the anterior maxillary region.
- The types that can be found are conical, also known as mesiodens, tuberculate, supplemental, and odontomes.

4.3.1.3 Early Loss of Deciduous Teeth

- There could be numerous reasons for early loss of deciduous teeth.
- Common causes could be caries, trauma, or root resorption.
- Early loss could result in crowding and space loss, which could possibly lead to impaction.
- For example, early loss of a lower deciduous E can result in mesial movement of the lower first molar, making no space for the lower premolar to erupt, resulting in impaction.

4.3.1.4 Extraction of Permanent Tooth

- Most commonly a first permanent molar.
- Extraction of a first permanent molar can result in crowding and space loss, which could possibly lead to impaction.
- Reasons for a first permanent tooth being extracted could be poor diet and oral hygiene, which can lead to caries.

4.3.2 Variation in Tooth Size

4.3.2.1 Macrodont

- A large tooth is known as a macrodont.
- This tooth will present with a large clinical crown.
- Macrodonts can be associated with supernumaries.
- A clinical feature that can result from macrodonts is dental crowding.

4.3.2.2 Microdont

- A small tooth is known as a microdont.
- This tooth will present with a small clinical crown.
- Microdonts can often be associated with hypodontia.
- A clinical feature that can result from microdonts is spacing.

4.3.2.3 Dento-alveolar Disproportion

- This is a term that relates to the teeth and jaws.
- Dento-alveolar disproportion is found when there is a mismatch in tooth and jaw size.
- For example, patients could present with big jaws but small (microdontia) teeth or small jaws and big (macrodontia) teeth.
- The clinical result that can be found with this is crowding or spacing.

4.3.2.4 Bolton Discrepancy

- This is an analysis which determines the size discrepancy between the size of the maxillary and mandibular teeth.
- It looks at the mismatch in tooth size and helps to analyse the optimum inter-arch relationship.
- Measurements are taken of the mesio and distal widths of all the teeth.
- This analysis was developed to achieve the ideal occlusion and inter-digitation.

4.3.3 Variation in Tooth Position

4.3.3.1 Infraocclusion (Ankylosis)

- Infraocclusion is also known as ankylosis.
- Ankylosis is when failure of eruption of a tooth occurs due to the anatomical fusion of cementum and alveolar bone.
- When a tooth is ankylosed, the tooth will submerge relative to its neighbours. It is important to know that when this happens the tooth is not sinking, its neighbouring teeth are erupting alongside the alveolar complex.
- The most commonly affected deciduous teeth are the first and second deciduous molars (Ds and Es).
- The most common cause of this is genetic and the condition has a high occurrence in patients with hypodontia.

4.3.3.2 Ectopic Tooth

- This is a term used to describe a certain type of eruption of a tooth.
- An ectopic tooth is a tooth that manages to erupt, but may erupt at an angle or in an aberrant position, rather than emerging in its correct position.

4.3.3.3 Impacted Teeth

- Impaction occurs when there is failure of eruption due to an obstruction such as tissue, bone, or another tooth.
- It occurs mostly when crowding is present.
- The most common teeth that are impacted are the upper canines (U3s), upper central incisors (U1s), and lower first permanent molars (L6s).

4.3.3.4 Transposition

- Transposition is a term used when the anatomical positions of teeth are interchanged.
- The most commonly affected teeth are the maxillary canines and first premolars and mandibular lateral incisors and mandibular canines.
- There are two types of transposition:
  - True transposition is found when the roots and crowns of the teeth have completely interchanged.
  - False transposition is found when the roots are in the correct position but the crowns have interchanged.

4.3.3.5 Primary Failure of Eruption

- This is seen when a tooth fails to fully erupt.
- It usually has a strong genetic basis.
- The most commonly affected teeth are the first and second permanent molars.

4.4 Habit

A thumb or finger sucking habit may exist until at least the age of 6–7 years. It can have a significant effect on occlusion, depending on the duration and intensity. Forces (intensity of the habit) acting more than six hours a day result in tooth movement such as:

- AOB
- Increased overjet
- Buccal crossbites.

4.5 Fraenal Attachments

4.5.1 Upper Labial Fraenum

- Patients who have a low fraenal attachment may present with a maxillary midline diastema.
- If the patient has an alveolar cleft between the incisors, a fraenectomy may be needed at the end of treatment.
- If the patient does not have a fraenectomy, this can result in the diastema reopening post-treatment.

4.5.2   Lower Labial Fraenum

A lower fraenal attachment can result in the following:

- Diastema
- Poor oral health
- Recession at the gingival margin.

5

Class I Malocclusion

5.1 Definition

The lower incisor edges occlude with or lie immediately below the cingulum plateau of the upper central incisors.

5.2 Prevalence

Fifty per cent of Caucasians present with this type of occlusion.

5.3 Aetiology of Class I

5.3.1 Skeletal Factors

- Patients can present with either a skeletal Class I, II, or III.
- They can present with dento-alveolar compensation, when they will have the following features:
  - Can be a skeletal II or III.
  - Skeletal II = upper incisors retroclined and lower incisors proclined.
  - Skeletal III = upper incisors proclined and lower incisors retroclined.
- Average, increased, or decreased lower anterior facial height (LAFH).
- Mandibular asymmetry or narrow maxilla can result in crossbites.

5.3.2 Soft Tissue Factors

- Patients usually have favourable soft tissues.
- They could present with bimaxillary proclination, a term used to describe the proclination of the upper and lower incisors.
- Features found with bimaxillary proclination are:
  - Weak muscular tone
  - Incompetent lips
  - Forward tongue position
  - Macroglossia tongue.

Textbook for Orthodontic Therapists, First Edition. Ceri Davies.
© 2020 John Wiley & Sons Ltd. Published 2020 by John Wiley & Sons Ltd.

5.3.3 Local Factors

- Dento-alveolar disproportion can result in crowding or spacing.
- Early loss of deciduous teeth can result in a centreline displacement.
- When there is crowding, teeth can become impacted, such as maxillary canines, maxillary central incisors, first permanent molars or premolars due to early loss of deciduous first molars (Ds) and secondary molars (Es).
- When there is spacing, the 'ugly duckling' stage can be seen when maxillary canines are not erupted. Once the canines have erupted this is usually self-correcting. Patients can present with a diastema due to:
  - Missing laterals
  - Microdont
  - Supernumerary
  - Low fraenal attachment
- Proclined incisors.

5.4 Treatment of Class I

There are five ways in which a class I malocclusion can be treated.

5.4.1 No Treatment

- Leave the malocclusion and accept the teeth, and their discrepancies, as they are.
- All patients must be informed of all the risks if they wish to take the no treatment option.

5.4.2 Removable Appliance

- Create space:
  - An upper removable appliance (URA) can be used to create space.
  - For example, distalization of the posterior segment can be achieved by the use of a nudger appliance with or without headgear.
- Maintain space:
  - A URA can be used as a space maintainer.
  - For example, its use in early loss of deciduous teeth will allow eruption of permanent teeth.
- Aligning:
  - A URA can be used to align the dentition by use of a labial bow.
  - Only tipping movements can be achieved with the use of URAs.
- Correct deepbite:
  - A URA can be useful for patients presenting with deepbites.
  - By incorporating a flat anterior bite plane (FABP) onto the URA, you can achieve incisor intrusion and passive lower molar eruption, which will help to open the patient's bite.

5.4.3 Fixed Appliance

- Extractions can be considered to relieve crowding in class I malocclusions:
  - Maxillary and mandibular second premolars for mild–moderate crowding.
  - Maxillary and mandibular first premolars for moderate–severe crowding.
  - Second premolars are considered for extractions if mild–moderate crowding is present. The reason they would be considered in this case is because extracting these teeth provides less space within the arch. However, first premolars are considered for moderate–severe crowding, as these provide more space anteriorly.
- Non-extractions can be considered for the following:
  - Self-ligating appliances.
  - Using an appliance that has low friction on the teeth.
  - Gaining upper arch expansion to create space, limiting the need for extraction.
  - Achieving a big wide smile creates space-enabling tooth alignment.

5.4.4 Headgear

Headgear can be used for the following reasons:

- Creating space:
  - Many different types of pull can be considered:
    - ○ Cervical low pull
    - ○ High pull
    - ○ Combi pull.
  - Creating space can be achieved by distalising the molars.
- Correcting a deepbite:
  - A cervical low pull would be considered.
  - This type of headgear pulls below the occlusal plane.
  - By pulling below the occlusal plane, distalisation of the molars and extrusion of the molars occur.
  - Extrusion of the molars helps to reduce the deepbite in the anterior region.

5.4.5 Surgery

Rapid maxillary expansion (RME) is used in the upper arch only. It consists of molar bands on U4s and U6s, with rigid arms extending from molar bands with a Hyrax screw. It achieves skeletal expansion by splitting the mid-palatine suture. Patients can activate the appliance up to four times a day by the use of a key, producing 1 mm of expansion movement a day. The appliance is left in situ for three months to allow for the bony infill of the mid-palatine suture (expanded suture).

6

Class II Div I Malocclusion

6.1 Definition

The lower incisor edges occlude posterior to the cingulum plateau of the upper central incisors. The upper central incisors are often proclined and there is an increased overjet.

6.2 Prevalence

Thirty-five per cent of Caucasians present with this type of occlusion.

6.3 Aetiology of Class II Div I

6.3.1 Skeletal Factors

- Patients will present with a skeletal Class II with retrognathic mandible.
- Dento-alveolar compensation:
  - Patients may be presenting with a skeletal Class II, however they could be presenting with class I incisors.
  - Patients who have retroclined upper incisors and proclined lower incisors are compensating for a class I incisor relationship; however, when these teeth have been decompensated patients will be turned into a class II div I malocclusion.
- Normal, increased or decreased lower anterior facial height (LAFH).

6.3.2 Soft Tissue Factors

- Patients could be presenting with incompetent lips for the following reasons:
  - They could be presenting with reduced coverage of the lower lip line, which results in proclined incisors.
  - Patients could present with a retrognathic mandible, resulting in incompetent lips. A retrognathic mandible is found when a patient presents with abnormal posterior positioning of the mandible. Another easier term used to describe this is a backwards positioning of the mandible (the mandible is sat further back relative to the maxilla).
  - Patients could be using excessive muscular activity, which is needed to achieve an oral seal.

Textbook for Orthodontic Therapists, First Edition. Ceri Davies.
© 2020 John Wiley & Sons Ltd. Published 2020 by John Wiley & Sons Ltd.

- Adaptive tongue thrust:
  - An adaptive tongue thrust is a tongue thrust that will cease once the incisors are in the correct position.
  - It is the habit of forcing the tongue between the teeth.
  - Common features found with a tongue thrust are an overjet and anterior open bite (AOB).
- Lower lip trap:
  - A lower lip trap can result in upper incisor proclination and lower incisor retroclination.
  - It is seen when the lower lip is drawn up behind the upper incisors.
- Strap-like lower lips:
  - Strap-like lower lips are also known as tight lips.
  - They cause retroclination of the lower incisors, making a class II div I look worse.
- Endogenous tongue thrust:
  - This is a tongue thrust that cannot be ceased once the teeth are in the correct position.
  - It is the habit of forcing the tongue between the teeth.
  - It can cause upper incisor proclination and AOB.
  - A patient with an endogenous tongue thrust will relapse once treatment is complete due to the habit continuing.

6.3.3   Local Factors

- Crowding:
  - Crowding can lead to incisors being proclined out of the arch labially, which can result in an increased overjet.
  - Teeth are pushed out of the arch due to there not being enough space for them.
- Spacing:
  - A diastema could be present.
  - This could be due to a digit sucking habit which has caused an increased overjet.
  - An underlying mesiodens may be present between the upper central incisors, erupted or unerupted.
- Anterior mandibular extractions:
  - Can lead to uprighting of the lower incisors under lip pressure and an increase in the overjet and overbite.

6.3.4   Habit

- A persistent digit sucking habit can cause:
  - Increased overjet
  - Narrow upper arch
  - Proclined upper incisors – class II div I
  - Low tongue position
  - Incomplete overbite
  - Retroclined lower incisors
  - Buccal crossbites.

6.4   Treatment of a Class II Div I

There are six ways to treat a class II div I malocclusion.

6.4.1   No Treatment

- Leave the malocclusion and accept the teeth and their discrepancies.
- All patients must be informed of the risks if they wish to take the no treatment option.

6.4.2   Removable Appliance

- Labial bow:
  - An upper removable appliance (URA) used with a labial bow incorporated.
  - This labial bow is used to retract the upper incisors, which will reduce an overjet.
  - When using a URA to reduce an overjet, it is important to make sure the acrylic which is positioned palatal to the upper anterior teeth is removed, if it is not the overjet will not reduce.
- Midline expansion screw:
  - A URA may be used with a midline expansion screw.
  - A class II div I case may present with buccal crossbites.
  - Expansion of the upper arch with a midline expansion screw will help to correct crossbites.
- Correct deepbite:
  - Patients could be presenting with a deepbite.
  - A URA can incorporate a flat anterior bite plane (FABP).
  - Incorporating this will allow passive lower molar eruption and lower incisor intrusion, which will help to open the deepbite.
- Create space:
  - Space may sometimes need creating.
  - Space can be created by incorporating two unilateral screws to help distalise the posterior segment.

6.4.3   Functional Appliance

A functional appliance may be any of these six appliances:

- Clark's twin block
- Herbst
- Bionator
- Medium opening activator (MOA)
- Clip-on fixed functional (COFF)
- Frankel.

A functional appliance postures the mandible forward, reducing the upper anterior segment and proclining the lower anterior segment to reduce the overjet.

6.4.4   Fixed Appliances

- Extractions can be considered to relieve crowding in class II div I malocclusions:
  - Maxillary first premolars only:
    - This is considered in a mild–moderate crowded case with a well-aligned lower arch.
    - In this case the maxillary first premolars are considered because more space is gained from these teeth; due to the need for more space anteriorly to reduce an overjet, this will help to retract the upper incisors.

- Maxillary first premolars and mandibular second premolars:
  o This is considered in a mild–moderate case with crowding in both arches.
  o Maxillary first premolars would be considered to help retract the upper incisors to reduce an overjet. These teeth are considered because more space is needed anteriorly for retraction.
  o Mandibular second premolars would be considered for moderate crowding on the lower arch, because less space is needed to align the dentition due to there only being mild–moderate crowding.
- Maxillary and mandibular first premolars:
  o This is considered in a moderate–severe crowded case in both arches.
  o Due to more space being needed in both arches, more space is gained by extracting the first premolars, therefore this would be a consideration in severe cases.
  o Mandibular first premolars are to be extracted if a patient has severe crowding in the lower arch.
- Intermaxillary elastics:
  - With a class II div I case, elastics will be considered.
  - Class II intermaxillary elastics would be used.
  - Class II elastics will help to retract the upper anterior segment and procline the lower anterior segment, which will help to reduce the overjet.
  - Class II elastics also work in our favour if a patient also presents with a deepbite, as this allows molar extrusion which will help to open the patient's bite.
- Space closure:
  - Fixed appliances will close all remaining spaces once the overjet has reduced.
  - For example, a patient has had upper first premolars and lower second premolars extracted. In the upper arch, lacebacks will be placed from the upper canines to the upper first permanent molars to achieve a class I canine relationship. Once the canines are in class I, chain elastic will be placed U2-2 to retract the remaining overjet. In the lower arch, lacebacks are used to relieve lower anterior crowding; once teeth are aligned the back teeth will be brought forwards (mesially) to close the remaining spaces.
- Correct deepbite:
  - A patient presenting with a deepbite can be corrected in this stage.
  - There are numerous ways of correcting a deepbite with fixed appliances:
    o Bond and engage 7s on archwire
    o Position anterior brackets more incisally
    o Reverse curve archwires
    o Composite/metal bite turbos
    o Fixed FABP
    o Clip-on FABP
    o Intermaxillary elastics – class II
    o Headgear – cervical low pull.
- Correct AOB:
  - A patient presenting with an anterior openbite can be corrected in this stage
  - There are a numerous ways of correcting a AOB with fixed appliances:
    o Posterior bite blocks – intrudes posterior segment
    o Positioning anterior brackets more gingivally
    o Reverse curve archwires (upside down)
    o Anterior box elastics

     ○ Incisor extrusion
     ○ Temporary anchorage devices (TADs)
     ○ Kim mechanics
     ○ Headgear – high pull.

6.4.5 Headgear

- Create space:
  - Headgear can be used to create space.
  - The type of headgear that would be used is the combi straight pull headgear.
  - This type of pull is level with the occlusal plane, which is used to distalise the maxillary molars.
- Correct deepbite:
  - Headgear can be used to correct a deepbite.
  - The type of headgear that would be used is the cervical low pull headgear.
  - This type of pull is below the occlusal plane, which is used to distalise and extrude the maxillary molars. By doing this it encourages a backward growth rotation, which will reduce the deepbite.
- Correct AOB:
  - Headgear can be used to correct an AOB.
  - The type of headgear that would be used is the high pull headgear.
  - This type of pull is above the occlusal plane, which is used to distalise and intrude the maxillary molars and achieve maxillary restraint. By doing this it encourages a forward growth rotation, which will reduce the AOB.

6.4.6 Surgery

Surgery can be given as a treatment option to some patients. The majority of patients who have surgery are severe cases. Patients presenting with a severe retrognathic mandible would be considered. The type of surgery would be a bilateral sagittal split osteotomy (BSSO), which achieves mandibular advancement.

7

Class II Div II Malocclusion

7.1   Definition

The lower incisor edges occlude posterior to the cingulum plateau of the upper central incisors.

The upper central incisors are retroclined and the overjet is minimal or increased. The common feature of this type of malocclusion is proclined laterals.

7.2   Prevalence

Ten per cent of Caucasians present with this type of occlusion.

7.3   Aetiology of Class II Div II

7.3.1   Skeletal Factors

Patients will present with a skeletal class II with a retrognathic mandible and with many features, such as:

- Reduced lower anterior facial height (LAFH) and Frankfort-mandibular plane angle (FMPA)
- Forward growth rotation
- High lower lip line
- Deepbite
- Pronounced labiomental fold.

A scissorbite may be seen in the premolar region due to a narrow lower arch.

7.3.2   Soft Tissue Factors

- High lower lip line:
  - Retroclination of the upper anterior segment can be seen if there is more than one-third coverage of the upper central incisors.
  - Lateral incisors have shorter crowns, which can escape the control of the lower lip and procline. The most common feature to be found with a class II div II malocclusion is proclined lateral incisors.

Textbook for Orthodontic Therapists, First Edition. Ceri Davies.
© 2020 John Wiley & Sons Ltd. Published 2020 by John Wiley & Sons Ltd.

- Labiomental fold:
  - The labiomental fold is found between the lower lip and the chin.
  - With a reduced LAFH, the labiomental fold will reflect the soft tissue lip abundance.
- Bimaxillary retroclination:
  - This term is used to describe the position of the upper and lower incisors.
  - Bimaxillary retroclination is where upper and lower incisors are retroclined due to a strap-like lower lip.

7.3.3 Local Factors

- Increased interincisal angle:
  - The interincisal angle is used when doing a cephalometric analysis.
  - This angle is located where the long axis of the upper and lower incisors meets.
  - The average value of the interincisal angle in Caucasians is $135°+/-10°$.
  - The interincisal angle can differ depending on the position of the incisors.
  - If the interincisal angle is reduced to its mean, then this suggests the patient is a class II div I.
  - If the angle has increased and is larger than its mean, then this suggests the patient is a class II div II; the reason it is larger is the retroclined upper and lower incisors.
- Gummy smile:
  - Due to retroclined upper central incisors, patients can be seen with a gummy smile.
  - This is a common feature with a class II div II case.
- Retroclined lower incisors:
  - Patients can have retroclined lower incisors.
  - This can be due to:
    o Deepbite, which can trap them.
    o Strap-like lips, which will retrocline them.
- Deep overbite:
  - A deep overbite can also have an effect on the position of the incisors:
    o Deep overbites can trap the lower incisors.
    o The position of the teeth can cause trauma to the palate and to the labial gingivae of the lower incisors from the upper incisors.
    o Can cause reduction of the intercanine width, which can cause a scissorbite in the premolar region.
- Crowding:
  - Crowding can be found within a class II div II case.
  - Retroclined incisors are often associated with this.
- Proclined or mesiolabial rotated lateral incisors:
  - This is a very common feature that is found within a class II div II case.
  - Causes of this can be:
    o Crowding
    o Failure of lower lip control.

7.4 Treatment of Class II Div II

There are six ways to treat a class II div II malocclusion.

7.4.1 No Treatment

- Leave the malocclusion and accept the teeth and their discrepancies as they are.
- All patients must be informed of all the risks if they wish to take the no treatment option.

7.4.2 Removable Appliance

- Anterior expansion screw or Z springs (double cantilever):
  - These are two active components which are found on a removable appliance.
  - Either component can be used to procline the incisors to turn them into a class II div I.
- Correct deepbite:
  - A flat anterior bite plane can be incorporated on the removable appliance to help reduce the deepbite.
  - This allows passive lower molar eruption and incisor intrusion.
- An alternative to a removable appliance is a sectional fixed U2–2 to turn the malocclusion into a class II div I.

7.4.3 Functional Appliance

- Any of these six appliances can be used:
  - Clark's twin block
  - Bionator
  - Herbst
  - Medium opening activator (MOA)
  - Clip-on fixed functional (COFF)
  - Frankel.
- These posture the mandible forward to reduce the upper anterior segment and procline the lower anterior segment to reduce the overjet.

7.4.4 Fixed Appliances

With class II div II cases, once the upper anterior teeth are proclined to their normal angulation, the patient will be turned into a class II div I case, where the overjet needs to be reduced.

- Extractions:
  - Maxillary first premolars only:
    o This is considered in a mild–moderate crowded case with a well-aligned lower arch.
    o In this case the maxillary first premolars are considered because more space is gained from these teeth. Due to the need for more space anteriorly to reduce an overjet, this will help to retract the upper incisors.
  - Maxillary first premolars and mandibular second premolars:
    o This is considered in a mild–moderate case with crowding in both arches.
    o Maxillary first premolars would be considered to help retract the upper incisors to reduce an overjet. These teeth are considered because more space is needed anteriorly for retraction.
    o Mandibular second premolars would be considered for moderate crowding in the lower arch, because less space is needed to align the dentition due to there only being mild–moderate crowding.

- Maxillary and mandibular first premolars:
  - o This is considered in a moderate–severe crowded case in both arches.
  - o Due to more space being needed in both arches, more space is gained by extracting the first premolars, therefore this would be a consideration in severe cases.
  - o Mandibular first premolars are to be extracted if a patient has severe crowding in the lower arch
- Intermaxillary elastics:
  - – With a class II div II case, elastics would be considered.
  - – Class II intermaxillary elastics would be used.
  - – Class II elastics help to retract the upper anterior segment and procline the lower anterior segment, which will help to reduce the overjet.
  - – In class II div II cases, patients present with deepbites. Class II elastics would work in our favour with this, as they allow molar extrusion, which will help to reduce the patient's deepbite.
- Space closure:
  - – Once the upper anterior teeth are in the correct inclination, the same class II div I procedures will apply to space closure.
  - – Fixed appliances will close all remaining spaces once the overjet has reduced.
  - – For example, a patient has had the upper first premolars and lower second premolars extracted. In the upper arch, lacebacks will be placed from the upper canines to the upper first permanent molars to achieve a class I canine relationship once the canines are in class I and the anterior segment has achieved its correct inclination, creating an overjet, and chain elastic will be placed U2–2 to retract the remaining overjet. In the lower arch, lacebacks are used to relieve lower anterior crowding, and once the teeth are aligned the posterior teeth will be brought mesially to close the remaining spaces.
- Correct deepbite:
  - – A patient in a class II div II will present with a deepbite, which can be corrected in this stage.
  - – There are numerous ways of correcting a deepbite with fixed appliances:
    - o Bond and engage 7s on archwire
    - o Position anterior brackets more incisally – this would work in the clinician's favour by positioning them incisally from the bond-up appointment
    - o Reverse curve archwires
    - o Composite/metal bite turbos
    - o Fixed FABP
    - o Clip-on FABP
    - o Intermaxillary elastics – class II
    - o Headgear – cervical low pull

7.4.5 Headgear

- Correct deepbite:
  - – Headgear can be used to correct a deepbite.
  - – The type of headgear that would be used is the cervical low pull headgear.
  - – This type of pull is below the occlusal plane, which is used to distalise and extrude the maxillary molars. By doing this it encourages a backward growth rotation, which will reduce the deepbite.

7.4.6 Surgery

Surgery can be given as a treatment option to some patients. The majority of patients who have surgery are severe cases. Patients presenting with a severe retrognathic mandible and deepbite would be considered. The types of surgery patients could have are:

- Mandibular segmental procedure:
  - This type of procedure would be done in a severe deepbite case.
  - This is where incisions are made lower 3–3 and the anterior segment is moved down to correct the deepbite.
- Bilateral sagittal split osteotomy (BSSO):
  - For mandibular advancement.
  - Done in patients with a retrognathic mandible, as it advances the mandible.

8

Class III Malocclusion

8.1   Definition

The lower incisor edges occlude anterior to the cingulum plateau of the upper central incisors. The overjet may be decreased or reversed.

8.2   Prevalence

Five per cent of Caucasians present with this type of occlusion.

8.3   Aetiology of Class III

8.3.1   Skeletal Factors

- Patients will present with a skeletal class III with severe cases showing a prognathic mandible.
- There are many reasons for patients to present with a skeletal class III base:
  - Increased mandibular length.
  - Forward positioning of the glenoid fossa.
  - Reduced maxillary length.
  - Short cranial base.
  - Reduced cranial base angle.
- There will be increased lower anterior facial height (LAFH) and Frankfort-mandibular plane angle (FMPA).
- Backward growth rotation will be present.
- A narrow maxilla or broad mandible can result in buccal crossbites.

8.3.2   Soft Tissue Factors

- Dento-alveolar compensation:
  - Found in the transverse dimension due to molars tipping lingually and palatally, compensating for a buccal crossbite.

Textbook for Orthodontic Therapists, First Edition. Ceri Davies.
© 2020 John Wiley & Sons Ltd. Published 2020 by John Wiley & Sons Ltd.

- Macroglossia tongue:
  - Also known as a large tongue.
  - The tongue appears to adopt lower than its normal resting position, which results in:
    ○ Broad lower arch
    ○ Posterior crossbites
    ○ Proclined lower incisors.

8.3.3 Local Factors

- Narrow upper arch
- Broad lower arch
- Crowding in upper arch
- Well-aligned or spaced lower arch
- Crossbites – posterior and anterior.

8.4 Treatment

There are six ways to treat a class III malocclusion.

8.4.1 No Treatment

- Leave the malocclusion and accept the teeth and their discrepancies.
- All patients must be informed of all the risks if they wish to take the no treatment option.

8.4.2 Removable Appliance

- Anterior crossbite:
  - Anterior expansion screw or Z springs incorporated into an upper removable appliance (URA).
  - Allows proclination by tipping the teeth labially to relieve anterior crossbites.
  - Posterior occlusal capping is needed to help open the bite to prevent any interferences that will stop the teeth from moving.
- Posterior crossbite:
  - Midline expansion screw or coffin spring incorporated into a URA.
  - Allows expansion by widening the upper arch to relieve posterior crossbites.
  - Posterior occlusal capping is needed to help open the bite to prevent any interferences that will stop the teeth from moving.
- Positive overjet:
  - Anterior expansion screw or Z springs incorporated into a URA.
  - Even though these springs help correct anterior crossbites, they also help to create a positive overjet.
- Anterior and posterior crossbites:
  - 3D expansion screw incorporated into a URA.
  - This allows expansion posteriorly and anteriorly to correct both types of crossbite.
  - Both screws will be turned on different days of the week.
  - Posterior occlusal capping is needed to help prevent any interferences that will stop the teeth from moving.

- Posterior occlusal cover:
  - Capping is found on the posterior segment of the URA.
  - This will disarticulate the occlusion to stop any occlusal interferences, allowing correction of crossbites.

8.4.3 Functional Appliances

- Functional appliances can be used with class III cases, although this is rare today.
  There are two types that can be used with class III patients:
  - Reverse Clark's twin block:
    o This is a two-piece functional appliance.
    o It works in roughly the same way as a Clark's twin block as used in a class II case; however, a slightly different rule applies.
    o The lower bite block comes behind the upper bite block to help retract the mandible.
    o It is rarely used in the UK.
  - Frankel Regulator III (FR3):
    o The appliance eliminates cheek pressure by the acrylic buccal shields and allows expansion.
    o It is rarely used.

8.4.4 Fixed Appliances

- Extractions are considered in a class III malocclusion to help align the teeth and correct the occlusion
  - Maxillary second premolars and mandibular first premolars:
    o These extractions would be considered in this case, as more space is required anteriorly in the lower arch to help retract the lower anterior segment.
    o More space is gained by extracting the first premolars, so this would be considered in the lower arch, which will help to create a positive overjet.
    o Maxillary second premolars would be considered if crowding in the upper arch is present.
  - Mandibular first premolars only:
    o This is considered when more space is required anteriorly in the lower arch to help retract the lower anterior segment – this approach is rarely used.
    o If a patient presents with a well-aligned upper arch, this type of extraction pattern may be considered.
  - Lower mandibular incisor:
    o This extraction pattern can be considered as it gains space in the lower anterior segment, which will help to retract the lower anterior segment.
    o This type of approach is rarely used.
    o Consideration of this extraction pattern may be given in adult patients who have severe recession or poor pathology on a lower incisor tooth.
- Intermaxillary elastics:
  - With a class III case elastics will be considered.
  - Class III intermaxillary elastics would be used.
  - Class III elastics will help to retract the lower anterior segment and procline the upper anterior segment, which will help to retract the lower arch to create a positive overjet.

- Round archwires:
  - Round archwires may be considered in the lower arch.
  - Use of round archwires only in the lower arch will help roll back the lower incisors.
  - If rectangular archwires are used, this will torque the lower anterior segment too much, which will make the class III look even worse and make it more difficult to correct.
- Crossbite elastics:
  - Most patients will present with buccal/posterior crossbites.
  - This is due to the broad lower arch.
  - Crossbite elastics can be used with fixed appliances to correct this.
  - Elastics will run from the palatal surface on the upper posterior teeth to the buccal surface of the lower posterior teeth.
  - These elastics achieve expansion, widening the upper arch to achieve correction.
- Space closure:
  - Space will be utilised from the start of treatment before the space is closed.
  - Lacebacks would be considered in the lower arch, which would help to retract the lower anterior teeth.
  - Once the canines are in a class I relationship, lacebacks would remain on the lower arch and chain elastic would be placed lower 2–2, which would help close the space by rolling back the lower anterior teeth for retraction.
  - When closing space on the upper arch, retraction of the upper teeth is not considered, as the lower teeth will be retracted to sit behind the upper teeth for a positive overjet.
  - Posterior teeth will be brought forward for space closure on the upper arch.
- Correct anterior open bite (AOB) if present:
  - A patient presenting with an AOB can be corrected in this stage.
  - There are a numerous ways of correcting an AOB with fixed appliances:
    - Posterior bite blocks to intrude the posterior segment
    - Positioning anterior brackets more gingivally
    - Reverse curve archwires (upside down)
    - Anterior box elastics
    - Incisor extrusion
    - Temporary anchorage devices (TADs)
    - Kim mechanics
    - Headgear – high pull.

8.4.5 Headgear

- High pull headgear:
  - This type of headgear is used to distalise molars, intrude molars, and for maxillary restraint.
  - It helps to correct an AOB by decreasing the LAFH by encouraging a forward growth rotation.
- Facemask:
  - This type of headgear is also known as reverse headgear.
  - It is used to move teeth mesially to close spaces (excess spaces) or to attempt to move the maxilla forward.
  - It is not commonly used.

8.4.6 Surgery

Surgery can be given as a treatment option to some patients. The majority of these patients who have surgery are severe cases. Patients presenting with a severe prognathic mandible would be considered. The types of surgery patients could have are:

- Bilateral sagittal split osteotomy (BSSO):
  - For mandibular retraction.
  - Done for patients with a prognathic mandible, as this will retract the mandible.
- Maxillary advancement:
  - Considered for maxillary advancement.
  - Done to achieve mesial movement on the maxilla.

9

Prevalences

Unless stated otherwise, these prevalences are based on values found in Caucasians.
Incisor relationship:

- Class I – 50%
- Class II div I – 35%
- Class II div II – 10%
- Class III – 5%

Cleft lip and palate:

- Cleft lip with or without cleft palate – 1 : 700 live births with a male : female ratio = 2 : 1
- Isolated cleft palate – 1 : 200 live births with a female : male ratio = 4 : 1

Anterior openbite (AOB):

- Caucasians – 2–4%
- African Caribbeans – 5–10%

Crossbite:
- 8–16%

Hypodontia:
- 6% of population and female : male ratio of 3 : 2

Commonly missing teeth:

- L5's – 3%
- U2's – 2%
- U5's – 3%
- L1's – 1%

Supernumeraries:

- 4% and male: female ratio of 2: 1
- Types of supernumeraries:
  - Conical – 75%
  - Tuberculate – 12%
  - Supplemental – 7%
  - Odontome – 6%

- Impacted canine:
  - 1–2%, female : male ratio 2 : 1
  - Palatally impacted canine: 85%
  - Buccally impacted canine: 15%

10

Hypodontia

10.1   Definition

Hypodontia is a word used to describe missing teeth. The term is used when there is congenital absence of one or more primary or secondary teeth.

10.2   Commonly Missing Teeth

In Caucasians the most common absent teeth within the dentition are:

- L5s = lower second premolars
- U2s = upper lateral incisors
- U5s = upper second premolars
- L1s = lower central incisors

   Wisdom teeth are also common missing teeth, however they do not come under hypodontia for the Index of Orthodontic Treatment Need (IOTN) criteria (see Chapter 33). Wisdom teeth are missing in 25% of the population.

   When looking at the most commonly missing teeth, it is normally a tooth at the end of the series, apart from the lower central incisors.

10.3   Prevalence of Hypodontia

In Caucasians:

- 6% of the population have hypodontia
- Females are more commonly affected than males at a ratio of 3 : 2

10.4   Prevalence of Missing Teeth

- L5s – 3%
- U2s – 2%
- U5s – 3%
- L1s – 1%

Textbook for Orthodontic Therapists, First Edition. Ceri Davies.
© 2020 John Wiley & Sons Ltd. Published 2020 by John Wiley & Sons Ltd.

10.5 Classifying Hypodontia

Hypodontia can be classified into mild, moderate, or severe cases:

- *Mild cases* would present with one to two missing teeth.
- *Moderate cases* would present with three to five missing teeth.
- *Severe cases* would present with six or more missing teeth.

10.6 Classifying Missing Teeth as a Whole

Other than hypodontia, there are two other terms that are used when describing missing teeth, depending on how many missing teeth there are:

- *Hypodontia*: fewer than six missing teeth.
- *Oligodontia*: more than six missing teeth.
- *Anodontia*: a total loss of teeth.

10.7 Aetiology of Hypodontia

The factors associated with the causes if hypodontia are:

Genetic factors:
- Family pattern/history of hypodontia.
- Not always necessarily the same tooth/teeth.

Local factors:
- Cleft lip and palate due to disruption in the dental lamina.

Syndromes:
- Down's syndrome.
- Hemifacial microsomia.

10.8 Medical Conditions Associated with Hypodontia

Some medical conditions can be associated with missing teeth, including:

- Cleft lip and palate
- Down's syndrome
- Ectodermal dysplasia (fangs)
- Anodontia (no teeth).

10.9 Factors Associated with Hypodontia

- *Delayed dental development*: on the lower arch the mandibular second premolars are the last teeth to form, followed by the maxillary second premolars. Radiographically these teeth are not visible until the age of 9, so it is important that their absence should be treated with care.

- *Microdontia*: peg laterals (Figure 10.1) can be seen with hypodontia and all small teeth, which is known as dento-alveolar disproportion.
- *Impacted canines*: impacted canines can occur due to missing laterals or microdontia laterals. This can happen because the canine uses the distal aspect of the lateral root for canine guidance for eruption. Without this, the canine can go off course and lead to impaction.
- *Abnormal tooth positions*: teeth can migrate into any available space, which can lead to tipping and rotation.
- *Transposition*: missing laterals can make the canine go off course and lead to transposition of the canine and first premolar.
- *Alveolar atrophy*: in hypodontia spaces alveolar bone shrinks, which makes tooth movement and implant placement in adult patients more difficult.
- *Retained deciduous teeth*: patients who have gone past the normal sequence of eruption of the second permanent dentition and still present with retained deciduous teeth should be taken with care (Figure 10.2). In the upper arch the upper second premolars are among the last teeth to erupt, which is usually around the age of 10 years, and for the lower around 11 years. Patients past the age of 13 presenting with retained deciduous molars should have radiographs taken (Figures 10.3–10.5) to locate the presence of the second premolars.

Figure 10.1 Missing UR2 with peg lateral.

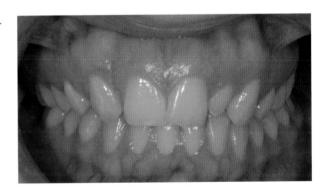

Figure 10.2 Upper occlusal intra-oral photograph showing missing U5s with retained deciduous molars (UEs).

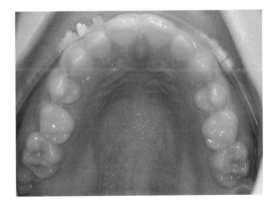

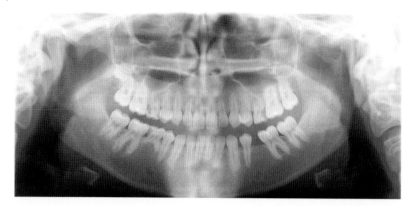

Figure 10.3 Dental panoramic tomograph showing all missing 5s and retained deciduous molars.

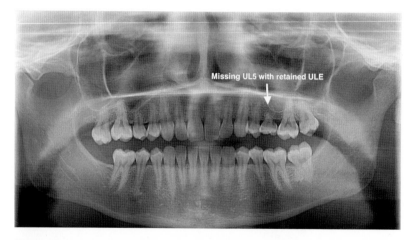

Figure 10.4 Dental panoramic tomograph showing missing upper left second premolar with retained deciduous molar.

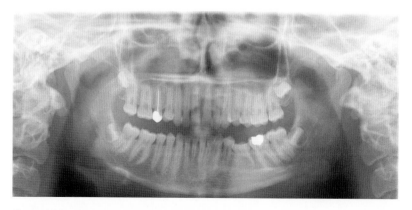

Figure 10.5 Dental panoramic tomograph of missing lower left second premolar (LL5) with retained deciduous molar (LLE).

10.10   Treatment of Hypodontia in Deciduous Teeth

Treatment of hypodontia in deciduous teeth is used mainly for psychological reasons. This can be in the form of a denture to help with and improve aesthetics and function.

10.11   Treatment of Hypodontia in Permanent Teeth

- *Second premolars*: two options can be considered when it comes to missing second premolars:
  - Close spaces and bring forward the first and second permanent molars (6s and 7s) and allow the wisdom teeth to erupt if present.
  - Open space for prosthetics such as an implant or a bridge.
- *Upper lateral incisors*: two options can be considered when it comes to missing upper lateral incisors (Figure 10.6):
  - Close spaces and modify the canine to look like a lateral incisor. Methods considered for this include:
    - ○ Invert the canine bracket. Canine roots are naturally positioned more labially, creating the buccal eminence, but inverting this bracket torques the root palatally.
    - ○ Place the canine bracket on the upper first premolar (U4s). This will torque the root labially, which is good for achieving buccal eminence.
    - ○ Place a lateral incisor (U2) bracket on the canine. This will change the torque of the canine tooth to make it look more like a lateral incisor.
    - ○ Build up the upper canines. At the end of treatment canines can be built up by the dentist to make them look more like lateral incisors.
  - Open space for prosthetics such as an implant or bridge.
    - ○ Once the patient has finished treatment, space needs to be maintained to prevent space closure of where the implant or bridge is going to be placed. Hawley retainers (Figure 10.7) can be modified to have a tooth-coloured pontic to maintain the space that has been created. Until the restorative work has been completed, the patient can wear the Hawley retainer full time, which means they will be less conscious of the gap and the pontic can be made to match to correct shade for the patient's teeth (Figure 10.8).

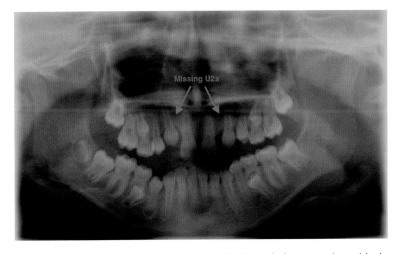

Figure 10.6   Dental panoramic tomograph showing missing upper lateral incisors.

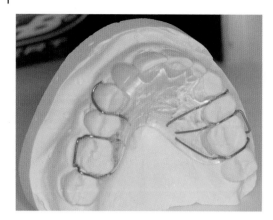

Figure 10.7 Hawley with pontic for UR2.

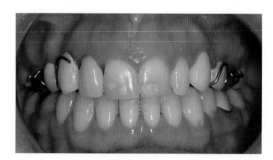

Figure 10.8 Hawley in situ with pontic for UR2.

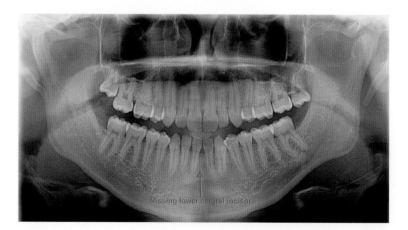

Figure 10.9 Dental panoramic tomograph showing missing lower central incisor.

- *Lower central incisors*: two options can be considered when it comes to missing lower central incisors (Figure 10.9):
  - Close space, especially in Class III, as it will help to retract lower teeth.
  - Open space for prosthetics such as an implant or bridge.

10.12   Implant Space Required

The space needed for an implant is 7 mm. However, during orthodontic treatment the orthodontist and the dentist who is doing the implant will liaise with each other to confirm the amount of space required. The dentist doing the implant must check they are happy with the amount of space before the appliance has been debonded so that, if necessary, the space can be adjusted.

10.13   Kesling Set-up

A Kesling set-up is used prior to treatment. It duplicates study models, which can show the patient the final aesthetic and occlusal outcome for closing or opening space.

11

Supernumeraries

11.1 Definition

A supernumerary tooth is an extra tooth. A supernumerary tooth is found when there are excess teeth in the normal series.

11.2 Prevalence of Supernumeraries

- Affect 4% of Caucasians.
- Males are twice as commonly affected as females.
- The most common area in which supernumeraries are found is the premaxilla region (80%).
- The second most common area is the mandibular premolar region.

11.3 Aetiology of Supernumeraries

- *Genetic factors*: there could be a family history of supernumeraries.
- Local factors: supernumeraries could be due to hyperactivity within the dental lamina.

11.4 Types of Supernumeraries

There are four types of supernumeraries:

- Conical, also known as mesiodens
- Tuberculate
- Supplemental
- Odontome.

11.5 Factors Caused by Supernumerary Teeth

There are two main factors that supernumerary teeth can cause:

- Displacement of erupted teeth.
- Impeded eruption, which can lead to impaction.

Textbook for Orthodontic Therapists, First Edition. Ceri Davies.
© 2020 John Wiley & Sons Ltd. Published 2020 by John Wiley & Sons Ltd.

11.6 Clinical Features of Supernumeraries

- Failure of eruption: supernumerary teeth can impede the eruption of surrounding teeth as they may lie in the path of the eruption.
- Diastema: a mesioden(s) present in the upper midline can cause a diastema.
- Crowding: an erupted supernumerary can take up arch space, resulting in crowding. Macrodont teeth are associated with supernumeraries.
- Displaced or rotated teeth.
- Root resorption of adjacent teeth.
- Cystic change within the follicle of the supernumerary.
- Prevention of tooth movement.

11.7 Medical Conditions Associated with Supernumeraries

Some medical conditions are associated with supernumeraries:

- Cleft lip and palate
- Cleidocranial dysplasia
- Gardner's syndrome.

11.8 Management of a Supernumerary

- Leave it and monitor if there is no orthodontic treatment. In this case the patient must have routine checks for any root resorption and cystic change.
- Extract and expose a permanent tooth if it is impacted.
- Extract to allow for orthodontic treatment.

11.9 Types of Supernumeraries

Conical, also known as mesiodens (Figures 11.1 and 11.2):

- Prevalence 75%.
- Most common supernumerary.
- Occurs in the premaxilla.
- Looks peg shaped.
- Termed mesiodens when found in the midline.
- Root formation is complete.

Tuberculate:

- Prevalence 12%.
- Barrel shaped.
- Consists of multiple tubercles.
- Occurs in the premaxilla.

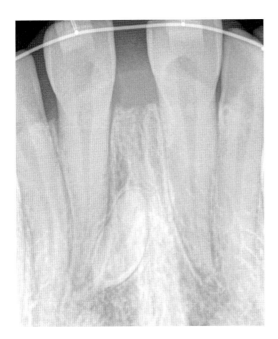

Figure 11.1 Upper occlusal standard radiograph. Unerupted mesiodens lying between roots of U1s.

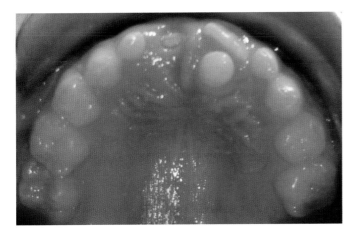

Figure 11.2 Upper occlusal intra-oral photograph. Mesioden erupting palatal to UL1.

- Is often paired.
- Forms palatal to upper central incisors.
- Can impede eruption of upper central incisors.
- Root formation is often incomplete.

Supplemental (Figures 11.3 and 11.4):

- Prevalence 7%.
- Resembles teeth of the normal series.
- Occurs at the end of a series.

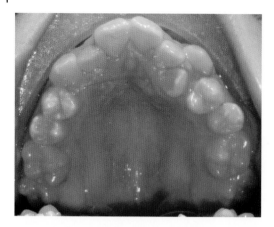

Figure 11.3 Upper occlusal intra-oral photograph showing supplemental tooth.

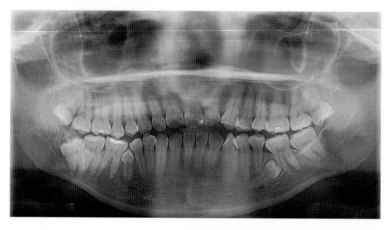

Figure 11.4 Dental panoramic tomograph showing supplemental tooth in the lower left quadrant.

- Most common area is the maxillary lateral incisor region.
- Second most common area is the mandibular premolar region.

Odontome (Figure 11.5):

- Prevalence 6%.
- Occurs rarely.
- Two types:
  - Complex: irregular mass of dental tissue.
  - Compound: well-organized tooth-like structure.
- Is a mass of tooth tissue.

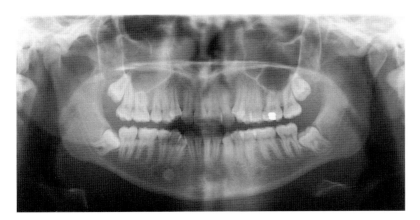

Figure 11.5   Dental panoramic tomograph showing odontome present around the lower right premolar region.

12

Impacted Canines

12.1 Definition

Impaction of a canine is where there is failure of eruption due to crowding or an obstruction within the dental arch. Obstruction could be due to crowding, a supernumerary, or fibrous tissue.

12.2 Prevalence of Maxillary Canines

- Affect 1–2% of Caucasians.
- Females are more commonly affected than males, with a ratio of 2 : 1.
- Prevalence of palatally positioned impacted canines is 85%.
- Prevalence of buccally positioned impacted canines is 15%.

12.3 Prevalence of Congenitally Missing Upper and Lower Canines

Total absence of missing upper and lower canines affects the Caucasian population with the following prevalences:

- Upper canines – 0.3%
- Lower canines – 0.1%.

12.4 Development of the Maxillary Canine

The maxillary canine begins its development high up in the maxilla at around the age of 4–5 months. The canine has a long path of eruption where it passes along the distal root surface of the lateral incisor and buccal to the deciduous canine, with eruption into its final position at around the age of 11–12 years. Canines should be palpable high in the buccal sulcus by the age of 10 years.

Textbook for Orthodontic Therapists, First Edition. Ceri Davies.
© 2020 John Wiley & Sons Ltd. Published 2020 by John Wiley & Sons Ltd.

12.5   Eruption of Upper and Lower Canines

The upper and lower canines erupt at different times:

- Upper canine eruption happens around the age of 11–12 years.
- Lower canine eruption happens around the age of 9–11 years.

12.6   Aetiology of Impacted Canine

- *Displacement of the crypt*: displaced crypts can result in severely displaced canines.
- *Long path of eruption*: the canine can go off course due to the long path of eruption.
- *Short-rooted or absent upper laterals*: the canines use the distal aspect of the lateral incisors to find their path. If they are absent or small, the canines can find it difficult to reach their destination.
- *Crowding*: not enough room for the canines can result in them being displaced buccally, palatally, or less commonly horizontally.
- *Retained deciduous canines*: these can result in the permanent canine losing its way because it is unable to erupt through its normal path.
- *Genetics*: studies show that impacted canines is an inherited trait.
- *Retention of primary deciduous canine*: the upper and lower maxillary canines usually erupt at around the age of 11 and 10 years, respectively. A patient 13+ years old presenting with retention of the primary deciduous canine will more than likely have an impacted canine.

12.7   Clinical Signs of an Impacted Canine

The following clinical signs can be seen on a patient who is presenting with an impacted canine:

- Canine is unable to be palpated in the buccal sulcus by the age of 10 years.
- Retained deciduous canines are sturdy and not mobile.
- There is a palatal bulge, which indicates the presence of the underlying canine.
- There is severe crowding and inadequate space within the dental arch, with not enough room for the eruption of canines.
- Increased mobility or non-vital maxillary central and lateral incisors could be an indicator of advanced root resorption of these teeth.

12.8   Radiographic Signs of an Impacted Canine

The following radiographic signs can be seen on the radiograph(s) of a patient who is presenting with an impacted canine:

- A palatal or buccal displaced canine using the parallax technique (see later discussion).
- The canine overlaps the lateral or central incisor root.
- The long axis of the canine is angled more than 25° to the vertical plane.

12.9 Parallax Technique for Radiographic Assessment of a Canine's Position

The parallax technique is used to assess and locate the position of an unerupted tooth or teeth.

It is most commonly used when a tooth needs to be located to find out its position and when it needs to be exposed.

There are two types of parallax, horizontal and vertical. Two views of the unerupted tooth are taken with the tube head in two positions. Assessing the direction the tooth has moved in relation to the tube head then identifies the position of the unerupted tooth.

The acronym SLOB is used for locating the position of an impacted canine:

- S – Same
- L – Lingual
- O – Opposite
- B – Buccal.

If the tooth moves in the *same* direction as the tube head of the X-ray, the tooth is positioned in a *lingual or palatal* position.

If the tooth moves in the *opposite* direction to the tube head, then the tooth is in a *buccal* position.

12.9.1 Horizontal Parallax

- Uses two periapical (PA) radiographs or two PAs and an upper standard occlusal radiograph.
- Horizontal parallax moves the tube head around the arch in the horizontal plane for each radiographic image. The tube head moves left and right.

12.9.2 Vertical Parallax

- Uses an orthopantogram (OPG) and an upper standard occlusal radiograph.
- Vertical parallax moves the tube head in the vertical plane, which changes the degree of angulation between the two radiographic images.
- The tube head on the dental panoramic tomograph (DPT) is aimed upwards at 8°.
- The tube head for an upper standard occlusal is aimed downwards at 65°.

In the example of vertical parallax in Figure 12.1, is the canine positioned lingually/palatally or buccally?

As Figure 12.2 shows, the canine is positioned lingually/palatally.

12.10 Management of Lingual/Palatal and Buccal Canines

12.10.1 Lingual/Palatal Canines: Surgical Exposure

- If the tooth is in a good position, then an open or closed surgical exposure, prior to orthodontic alignment, is considered to allow for the tooth to be extruded into the correct position.
  - Open exposure (Figure 12.3):
    - The canine is uncovered by removing bone and the overlying soft tissue.
    - Packing is placed in the exposure to prevent it from closing.

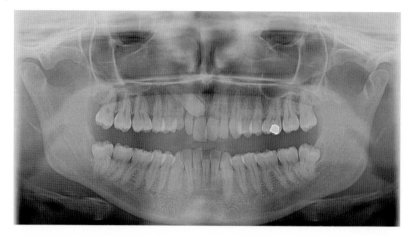

Figure 12.1 Digital panoramic tomograph showing impacted upper right canine.

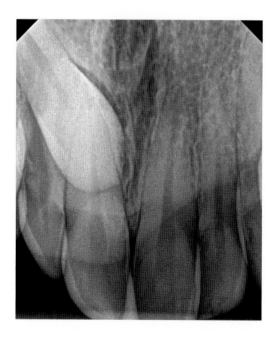

Figure 12.2 Upper standard occlusal radiograph of impacted upper right canine. The canine is positioned lingually/palatally.

- o Once the procedure has been completed, the patient must return to the orthodontic practice to have an attachment placed onto the tooth before it closes. If the patient does not come back in time, there is a risk of the exposure closing and the procedure needing to be redone.
  - Closed exposure (Figure 12.4):
    - o The canine is uncovered and an attachment with a gold chain is placed on the tooth surface; the gum is then stitched back over the tooth. The tooth can be pulled through the soft tissue via the gold chain.

Figure 12.3 Upper occlusal intra-oral radiograph: open exposure.

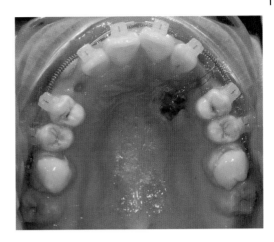

Figure 12.4 Upper occlusal intra-oral radiograph: closed exposure.

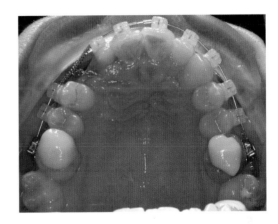

12.10.2 Buccal Canines

- Treatment may differ from palatally positioned canines.
- Patients may have orthodontic treatment first to create space to see if the canine will spontaneously erupt itself, as buccal canines have more of a chance of eruption due to the thin mucosa and bone on the buccal surface.
- This is usually done for about six months.
- If this does not work, surgical exposure is needed.

12.10.3 Surgical Removal

This is advised when:

- The canine is in a very unfavourable position due to the risk of root resorption to adjacent teeth if it is left.
- Patients are poorly motivated.
- There is severe crowding.

12.10.4 Auto Transplantation

- This involves surgical removal of an impacted canine and implantation of this tooth into its normal position within the maxillary alveolus.
- Space needs to be created to accept the transplant.
- It is not commonly done due to the risk of ankylosis.

12.11 Dressings for Open Exposure

Two types of dressing can be used to pack an open exposure:

- COE-PAK™ (GC Europe, Leuven, Belgium)
- Gauze.

12.12 Risks of Impacted Canines

12.12.1 Resorption

- Resorption is the biggest risk associated with impacted canines.
- The clinical crown of the canine can go off course and start to resorb the root of an adjacent tooth, most commonly the lateral incisor.
- If the canine lies 25° to the vertical plane, then action must be taken to protect the adjacent teeth.

12.12.2 Transposition

- Canines can go off course and erupt, most commonly between the premolars.
- If the canine has erupted nicely, then orthodontic treatment can commence to mask the premolar into a canine and the canine into a premolar by restorative work.

12.13 Position of Impacted Canines

- If a canine is more *vertically positioned* there is a *good* chance of it coming down.
- If a canine is *horizontally positioned* there is *not* a good chance of it coming down.

However, it all depends:

- If the canine is positioned more to the mid-sagittal plane, there is less of a chance of the canine coming down, depending on how high it is placed.
- An increased angle of >25° results in a horizontal canine which cannot come down.
- An average angle of 25° results in a vertical canine which can come down.

12.14 Ankylosis

- Ankylosis is the biggest risk that can occur with surgical exposure of a canine.
- Before surgical exposure, ankylosis of the canine cannot be seen. It is only when there has been no improvement in the position of canine that it is termed ankylosed.

- Ankylosis of a canine can be seen during orthodontic treatment when there is no improvement of the canine coming down.
- The following features can be seen when a canine is ankylosed:
  - When two DPTs are compared, a canine that appears in the same position on a radiograph a good 6–12 months after exposure.
  - No sign of the tooth erupting through the gum.
  - Intrusion of the adjacent teeth.
  - Archwire that is still bowed and appears to be still active if it is placed through the gold links of the exposure.
  - Ligature that has not become loose and appears still to be active.
  - No removal of gold chain links indicates no movement of canine.

13

Impacted Teeth

13.1 Definition

Impaction of a tooth is where there is failure of eruption due to crowding or an obstruction within the dental arch. Obstruction could be due to crowding, a supernumerary, or fibrous tissue.

13.2 Common Impacted Teeth

- Maxillary canines (see Chapter 12)
- Mandibular canines
- Maxillary central incisors
- Premolars
- First permanent molars
- Third permanent molars.

13.2.1 Impacted Mandibular Canines

- These teeth are less commonly impacted than maxillary canines.
- Impaction can be due to crowding.
- If space is available, these teeth can erupt spontaneously due to being vertically orientated and labially placed.
- If these teeth need to be surgically exposed, they should erupt through the attached gingivae.
- If the mandibular canines are orientated horizontally, they can fail to erupt.
- There are other treatment options for these teeth other than surgical exposure, such as extraction or auto transplantation.

13.2.2 Impacted Maxillary Central Incisors

- Prevalence of 0.13% in Caucasians.
- The aetiology of impaction of these teeth can be due to a supernumerary tooth such as a tuberculate, a retained deciduous incisor, or dilaceration.

Textbook for Orthodontic Therapists, First Edition. Ceri Davies.
© 2020 John Wiley & Sons Ltd. Published 2020 by John Wiley & Sons Ltd.

- Confirming this tooth is impacted should be done with care. If the opposing maxillary central incisor and lateral incisor have erupted six months prior to the central incisor, this can be termed impacted.

Management:

- The amount of space that is needed must be the correct space to allow for extrusion of the impacted tooth. The average size of the incisor is around 9 mm.
- Many cases of impaction of a maxillary central incisor can be due to supernumeraries such as a tuberculate and possibly a mesiodens. If this is the case these obstructions must be removed.
- Before considering surgical exposure, a space maintainer could be fitted to see if this tooth will erupt spontaneously.
- If there is no spontaneous movement, surgical exposure is considered.

13.2.3 Impacted Premolars

- The most common premolars that become impacted are the second premolars.
- The reason for impaction could be early loss of the second deciduous molar and mesial movement of the first permanent molar, which results in space loss for the second premolar to erupt.
- A supplemental supernumerary in the premolar region can also cause impaction to the second premolar.

Management:

- To allow eruption of the second premolars, extraction of the first premolars can be considered.
- By distalising the first permanent molars, space will be created to allow eruption of the second premolars.
- In cases where both dental arches are well aligned, extraction of the second permanent molars can be considered. The aim of doing this is to achieve spontaneous distal movement of the first permanent molars, which will allow space for the second premolars to erupt.

13.2.4 Impacted First Permanent Molars

- Prevalence is between 0.75% and 6%.
- More commonly seen in males than in females.
- Maxillary molars are the most common molar to be impacted.
- The aetiology of impaction to these teeth is due to crowding, ectopic positioning of the first molar crypt, and unfavourable crown positioning of the second deciduous molar.
- Risks that can occur to impacted first permanent molars include:
  - Root resorption of the deciduous molar, resulting in loss of vitality.
  - Loss of space in the dental arch.
  - Caries occurring to the first permanent molar due to this area being hard to clean.

Management:

- Observing the tooth:
  - Observation for spontaneous movement for three to six months.
  - If no improvement then treatment is considered.

- Separating the tooth:
  - Need to move the first permanent molar distally.
  - Achieved by use of a metal separator known as a brass wire.
  - Inserted by the contact point of the mesial aspect of the first permanent molar.
  - Inserted by use of lightwire pliers.
  - Tightened once a week to ensure equal force.
- If second permanent molars are erupted:
  - Upper removable appliance (URA) with palatal finger springs to distalise the second permanent molars.
  - Headgear to distalize the second permanent molars.
  - Fixed appliances with a transpalatal arch (TPA) to prevent mesial movement.
  - All to make space for the first permanent molars.
- Extraction:
  - Only considered if there is severe root resorption of second deciduous molars.
  - The risk is that this can result in space loss and crowding in the premolar region.

13.2.5 Impacted Third Permanent Molars

- Prevalence is 30–50% of Caucasians.
- Mandibular third molars are the most commonly affected.
- Aetiology of impaction can be due to:
  - Crowding
  - Ectopic positioning (abnormal position).
- Impacted wisdom teeth are associated with the following risks:
  - Root resorption of the second permanent molar
  - Caries
  - Swollen gum in the area of the wisdom tooth (pericoronitis)
  - Cysts found around teeth due to infection or trauma from the impaction.
- There are two treatment options for impacted wisdom teeth:
  - If the impacted wisdom teeth are not causing any harm to the patient, they can be left, but are monitored closely at regular check-ups.
  - If the teeth are causing the patient problems, their removal is considered.
- Risks of removing wisdom teeth:
  - Wisdom teeth removal is not a straightforward procedure and can lead to the following risks:
    o Inferior alveolar and lingual nerve damage, when patients can be left feeling numb and have no sensation due to the nerve being damage on removal.
    o Infections during and after removal.
    o Risks if putting patients under general anaesthesia.
  - Dentists can remove wisdom teeth in the dental chair. However, depending on the position of the impacted wisdom teeth, sometimes patients need to be referred to hospital to have them removed under general anaesthetic due to the tooth being positioned too close to the nerve.
- If the patient is currently in a fixed appliance and the wisdom teeth are partially erupted, bonding brackets on these teeth can be considered to help align them.

14

Deepbites

14.1 Definition

A deepbite is the vertical overlap of the upper incisors over the lower incisors when the posterior segment is in occlusion, where the upper incisors overlap the lower incisors by 4 mm or more.

14.2 Classifying Overbites

When classifying overbites, the lower incisors are visually divided into thirds, which will help to classify a patient's overbite as normal, increased, or decreased. As well as looking at this, the patient's overbite is then described as either complete or incomplete. This refers to whether the patient bites onto hard or soft tissue or not at all when they are in occlusion.

- Normal (Figure 14.1): the upper incisors cover one-third of the lower incisors with the posterior segment in occlusion.
- Increased (Figure 14.2): the upper incisors cover more than one-third of the lower incisors when the posterior segment is in occlusion.
- Decreased (Figure 14.3): the upper incisors cover less than one-third of the lower incisors when the posterior segment is in occlusion.
- Incomplete (Figures 14.4 and 14.5): the lower incisors do not come into contact with hard or soft tissues.
- Complete (Figures 14.6 and 14.7): the lower incisors do come into contact with hard or soft tissues.

14.3 Aetiology of a Deepbite

14.3.1 Skeletal Factors

- *Skeletal II pattern*: the mandible is retruded (set back) relative to the maxilla. This is known as mandibular retrognathia.
- *Reduced lower anterior facial height* (LAFH) due to the mandibular symphysis curving more anteriorly.

Textbook for Orthodontic Therapists, First Edition. Ceri Davies.
© 2020 John Wiley & Sons Ltd. Published 2020 by John Wiley & Sons Ltd.

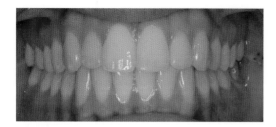

Figure 14.1 Normal overbite.

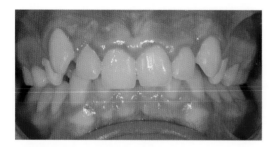

Figure 14.2 Increased overbite.

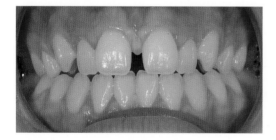

Figure 14.3 Decreased overbite.

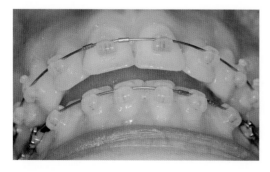

Figure 14.4 Incomplete overbite.

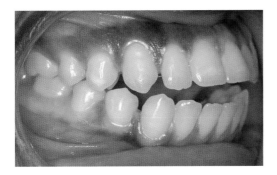

Figure 14.5 Incomplete overbite.

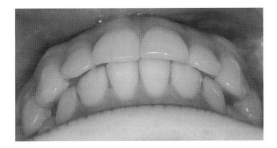

Figure 14.6 Complete overbite.

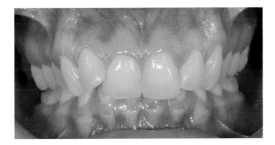

Figure 14.7 Complete overbite.

- *Forward growth rotation* due to vertically inclined condyle and mandibular symphysis, which can lead to upright or retroclined lower incisors.

14.3.2 Soft Tissue Factor

- *High lower lip line*: the lower lip covers more than one-third of the upper incisors, causing retroclination of the upper central incisors, which increases the interincisal angle.

14.3.3 Local Factor

- *Poorly formed cingulum plateau*: no positive occlusal stop at the cingulum plateau results in the lower incisors erupting past this point, which increases the overbite and the interincisal angle.

14.4 Treating Deepbites

There are five ways in which a deepbite can be treated.

14.4.1 Removable Appliance

A flat anterior bite plane (FABP) disarticulates the posterior segment and the lower anterior incisors only make contact on the bite plane. This allows incisor intrusion and passive lower molar eruption, which help to reduce the deepbite.

14.4.2 Functional Appliance

This results in posterior open bites (POB) at the end of treatment, which reduces the deepbite by the acrylic bite blocks (Clark's twin blocks) that are incorporated within the appliance and because of forward posturing of the mandible. A medium opening activator (MOA) helps to reduce the deepbite due to the lack of molar capping.

14.4.3 Fixed Appliance

There are many different techniques that can be used with fixed appliances when correcting deepbites. These include:

- Bond and engage second permanent molars (7s), which will increase the wedge effect.
- Reverse curve archwires to allow incisor intrusion and molar extrusion.
  - When positioning the lower archwire, it will go above the brackets on the posterior segment and under the brackets on the anterior segment on insertion.
  - Depending on how much upper incisor is showing when the patient smiles, this archwire can be placed in the upper arch. If the upper archwire is to be used, the archwire will be placed differently and will go below the brackets on the posterior segment and above the brackets on the anterior segment on insertion.
- Composite/metal bite turbos allow incisor intrusion and molar extrusion.
- A fixed FABP allows incisor intrusion and molar extrusion.
- A clip-on FABP also allows incisor intrusion and molar extrusion.
- Class II intermaxillary elastics will achieve molar extrusion.

14.4.4 Headgear

- A cervical low pull will distalise and extrude the molars.
- Encouraging a backward growth rotation and increasing the LAFH by extrusion of the posterior segment will reduce the deepbite by increasing the wedge effect.
- The force transmitted is below the occlusal plane.

14.4.5 Surgery

This option could be considered for some patients who have a severe deepbite that needs surgery for correction. The surgery procedures considered are:

- Mandibular segmental procedure:
  - This is where incisions are made to move the lower labial segment down.
  - Doing this will help to reduce the deepbite.
- Bilateral sagittal split osteotomy (BSSO):
  - A severe retrognathic mandible could be making the deepbite severe.
  - This procedure will achieve mandibular advancement, which will help to improve and reduce the deepbite.

14.5   Stability of a Deepbite

- *Growth*: young patients who are still likely to grow and have had their deepbite corrected are likely to have a relapse if there is forward growth rotation.
- *Positive occlusal stop*: at the end of treatment it is important to ensure that there is a positive occlusal stop at the cingulum plateau, as this will prevent the lower incisors from erupting past it, which can result in a deepbite.
- *Inter-incisal angle*: ensure that this is $135° \pm 10°$.

15

Openbites

Anterior and Posterior

Anterior openbite (AOB) and posterior openbite (POB) are terms used to describe two types of openbite.

15.1 Definition of an AOB

An AOB is found where there is no vertical overlap of the upper and lower incisors when the posterior segment is in occlusion.

15.2 Prevalence of AOBs

The prevalence of AOBs varies within the population:

- 2–4% of Caucasians
- 5–10% of African Caribbeans.

15.3 Classification of AOBs

An AOB can be classified into three types:

- *Mild* (Figure 15.1): an AOB is classified as mild if it is open between 1 and 2 mm.
- *Moderate* (Figure 15.2): an AOB is classified as moderate if it is open between 2 and 4 mm.
- *Severe* (Figure 15.3): an AOB is classified as severe if it is open more than 4 mm.

15.4 Aetiology of an AOB

Causes of an AOB are categorised into different types of factors.

Textbook for Orthodontic Therapists, First Edition. Ceri Davies.
© 2020 John Wiley & Sons Ltd. Published 2020 by John Wiley & Sons Ltd.

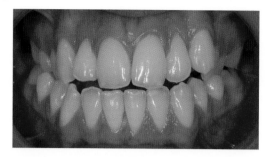

Figure 15.1 Mild anterior openbite.

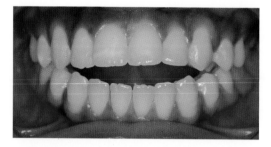

Figure 15.2 Moderate anterior openbite.

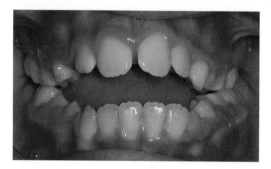

Figure 15.3 Severe anterior openbite.

15.4.1 Skeletal Factors

- *Skeletal III pattern*: this is due to an increased lower anterior facial height (LAFH).
- *Backward growth rotation*: this type of growth rotation has an anteriorly inclined mandibular symphysis, which leads to an increased LAFH and a greater chance of an AOB.
- *Condylar resorption*: resorption of the condyle can be due to mandibular trauma, which can affect the condyle itself. If this happens, resorption can result in the mandible being pulled backwards and downwards, resulting in an AOB.

15.4.2 Soft Tissue Factors

- *Forward tongue position*: intrusion of the incisors can occur from the position and pressure of the tongue, which causes an AOB.

- *Adaptive or endogenous tongue thrust*: a feature of this type of tongue thrusts is that the tongue gets thrusted forward when the patient swallows due to there being no anterior oral seal. This applies intrusive and proclining force to the teeth, which increases the chance of an AOB.
- *Macroglossia tongue*: a large tongue can result in an AOB.
- *Chronic nasal obstruction*: patients who have enlarged adenoids need to breathe through their mouth. Due to this, an AOB can occur as the molars can over-erupt. This is mainly seen in patients who are going through puberty, as after puberty the adenoids disappear.
- *Reduced muscular tone*: muscular dystrophy is due to reduced muscular tone (muscle weakness). Patients who are likely to have this will present with an increased LAFH with an AOB. This is because the low muscular tone allows the teeth to move freely due to less pressure from the soft tissues.

15.4.3 Local Factor

- *Cleft lip and palate*: this can result in teeth not erupting and prevent the archform from developing, because of which it may result in an AOB.

15.4.4 Habit

- *Digit sucking habit*: a constant intrusive force to the incisors can result in an AOB and also change the archform.

15.5 Treatment of an AOB

There are four ways to treat an AOB:

15.5.1 Removable Appliance

Posterior bite blocks can help in patients who are presenting with an AOB, as they intrude the posterior segment, which decreases the wedge effect, reducing the AOB.

15.5.2 Fixed Appliances

Different techniques can be used to help reduce an AOB with the use of fixed appliances:

- *Posterior bite blocks* (made of glass ionomer cement or GIC) intrude the posterior segment.
- *Anterior box elastics* extrude the upper and lower anterior segments.
- *Upside-down reverse curve archwires* intrude molars and extrude incisors.
  - The lower archwire on insertion goes below the brackets on the posterior segment and above the brackets on the anterior segment.
  - The upper archwire on insertion goes above the brackets on the posterior segment and below the brackets on the anterior segment.
- *Bracket positioning*: the brackets are positioned more gingivally to extrude the incisors and more occlusally to intrude the posterior segment. The disadvantage of this is that the procedure can be unstable and there is a change in the gingival margin.

- Temporary anchorage devices (TADs) are used to help intrude the posterior segment.
- *High pull headgear* would be used to distalise and intrude molars and achieve maxillary restraint.
- *Kim mechanics*: this is not a common technique used today but is an option that can be considered. It is used in conjunction with TADs, which are placed on the buccal and palatal surfaces. An elastic is then used which runs from both of the TADs. A transpalatal arch is also used to prevent flaring of the molars and keep the intermolar width.

15.5.3 Headgear

High pull headgear is considered for correction of an AOB. This will:

- Achieve distalisation of molars, intrusion of molars, and maxillary restraint.
- Transmit force above the occlusal plane.
- Encourage a forward growth rotation and, by intruding the posterior segment, decrease the LAFH and wedge effect, which reduces the AOB.

15.5.4 Surgery

Two types of surgery can be considered in severe AOB cases:

- *Le Fort I*: this type of surgery is done by moving the maxilla downwards.
- *Bilateral sagittal split osteotomy* (BSSO): this type of surgery moves the mandible into the correct position:
  - In Class II cases with an AOB – mandibular advancement.
  - In Class III cases with an AOB – mandibular setback.

15.6 Factors That May Make Stability of an AOB Poor

- *Backward growth rotation*: young patients who have more growth post-orthodontic treatment have the risk of relapse due to this increasing the LAFH and producing an AOB again.
- *Forward tongue position*: patients who have a forward tongue position that is still present post-orthodontic treatment have the risk of relapse, as this can result in intrusion to the incisors, which can lead to an AOB due to the pressure of the tongue.

15.7 Definition of a POB

A POB can be found when there is no vertical overlap of the upper and lower posterior teeth when the posterior segment teeth are in occlusion (Figure 15.4).

15.8 Facts about POBs

- They occur more rarely than AOBs.
- Early extraction of the first permanent molars can lead to a POB due to the possibility of a lateral tongue spread that could cause this.

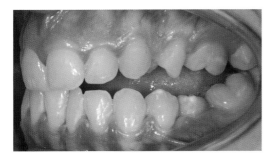

Figure 15.4 Posterior openbite.

- Cases where there are submerged teeth on the buccal segments can result in a POB.
- POBs could also be a result of an AOB that has extended posteriorly.

15.9 Aetiology of an POB

15.9.1 Primary Failure of Eruption

- This is found where the molars do not erupt.
- Extraction of these teeth is one of the treatment alternatives considered.

15.9.2 Arrest of Eruption

- This is found when the first molars begin to erupt according to their normal course of eruption, but for some reason stop.

15.9.3 Infraoccluded or Ankylosed Deciduous Teeth

- POBs can occur due to infraoccluded (submerged) deciduous teeth. Infraoccluded teeth are found when the surrounding teeth are continuing to erupt vertically, but the submerged tooth is left behind. It appears as though the infraoccluded tooth is sinking, but it is not as its neighbours are growing vertically. This can be seen when early loss of the second deciduous molar occurs and the first premolar and first permanent molar erupt, but tilt in towards each other. This obstructs the second premolar from erupting, even though it is not ankylosed, which is also known as submergence.
- Ankylosis is a term that is used when the tooth is fused to the bone and does not fully erupt. Ankylosed teeth do not respond to orthodontic forces, as there is no periodontal ligament around the tooth.

15.9.4 POBs Occurring from Twin Blocks

- Functional appliance treatment using twin blocks can result in POBs.
- This is due to forward posturing of the mandible in class II cases and the acrylic bite blocks, which cause intrusion to the posterior segment.

15.10   Treatment of POBs

15.10.1   Fixed Appliances

There are a few different techniques that can be used with this type of appliance:

- Posterior box elastics:
    - The elastic is attached to four teeth, two on the upper arch and two on the bottom, forming the shape of a box.
    - This helps to bring the teeth together and touching, closing any POB.
- Zigzag elastics:
    - These elastics are attached to a few teeth on the posterior segment.
    - They help to bring the teeth together during the finishing stages.
    - They form the shape of a zigzag.
- Posterior V elastics:
    - These elastics attach to three teeth and form the shape of a V.
    - They help bring the teeth together and touching.
    - They can be used on anterior teeth or posterior teeth.

16

Crossbites

16.1 Definition

A crossbite is found when there is an abnormal relationship between the opposing teeth in a bucco-palatal or bucco-lingual direction.

16.2 Types of Crossbites

Three types of crossbites can be found:

- *Posterior crossbite* (also known as a buccal crossbite; Figure 16.1): the **b**uccal cusps of the lower teeth occlude **b**uccal to the **b**uccal cusps of the upper teeth (BBB) when the patient is in full occlusion.
- *Anterior crossbite* (Figure 16.2): one or more of the maxillary incisors occludes lingual to the lower incisors, with the posterior teeth in occlusion.
- *Lingual crossbite/scissorbite* (Figure 16.3): the **b**uccal cusps of the lower teeth occlude **p**alatal to the **p**alatal cusps of the upper teeth (BPP) when the patient is in full occlusion.

16.3 Prevalence of Crossbites

Crossbites affect the Caucasian population at a prevalence of between 8 and 16%.

16.4 Crossbites That Can Occur

Crossbites can be found either on one side of the arch, known as unilateral, or on both sides, known as bilateral. Displacements can also occur when a crossbite is present. A displacement is found when the teeth on route to occlusion meet an interference (such as a crossbite). Due to this interference, the teeth then work around this to achieve maximum digitation. This can be seen where the patient slides their mandible into a more comfortable position.

Textbook for Orthodontic Therapists, First Edition. Ceri Davies.
© 2020 John Wiley & Sons Ltd. Published 2020 by John Wiley & Sons Ltd.

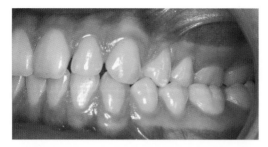

Figure 16.1 Posterior crossbite on UL7, UL6, and UL5, with buccal crossbite tendency on UL4.

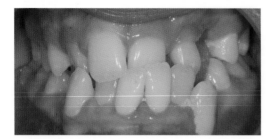

Figure 16.2 Anterior crossbite on UL1, UL2, and UR2, with poor oral hygiene.

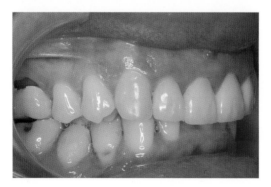

Figure 16.3 Lingual crossbite (scissorbite) present on UR4.

Crossbites that can occur are:

- Unilateral buccal crossbite with displacement
- Unilateral buccal crossbite with no displacement
- Bilateral buccal crossbite
- Unilateral lingual crossbite
- Bilateral lingual crossbite.

16.5 Aetiology of a Crossbite

16.5.1 Skeletal Factors

- *Skeletal class III cases*: due to the mandible being set forward relative to the maxilla, buccal cross-bites can be found. The most common type of crossbite in skeletal III cases is an anterior crossbite.

- *Skeletal class II cases*: due to the mandible being set back relative to the maxilla, lingual crossbites can be found. Patients with a digit sucking habit can also present with a posterior crossbite.
- *Narrow maxilla*: patients who have a narrow maxilla can present with a unilateral or bilateral buccal crossbite. This is due to the mismatch in arch size and form. It is also seen in patients with a digit sucking habit, as the pressure from the habit can narrow the upper arch, resulting in a buccal crossbite.
- *Mandibular displacement*: deviation of the mandible on closure for maximum interdigitisation can result in a unilateral crossbite.

16.5.2 Soft Tissue Factor

- *Chronic nasal obstruction* leads to a stuffy nose.
  - This may result in a buccal crossbite due to narrowing of the maxilla.
  - Mouth breathing can lead to a change of position of the tongue from its normal resting place in the palate. The change in the tongue position can alter the balance of forces between the tongue and the cheeks, which also results in a narrow maxilla.

16.5.3 Local Factors

- *Dental crowding* is the most common cause of crossbites.
  - Lateral incisors are the most common teeth to be crowded, which can result in an anterior crossbite.
  - If early loss of the second deciduous molars occurs, the second premolars are also frequently crowded, which can result in a crossbite.
  - Crowding can cause displacement of erupted/erupting teeth in the permanent dentition, which can result in a crossbite.
- *Cleft lip and palate*, which occurs when the palatal shelves of the palate fail to fuse together when they go from a vertical to horizontal position around the eighth week of intra-uterine life (see Chapter 36).
  - Crossbites appearing with a cleft lip and palate are due to the upper arch being narrow relative to the lower arch.
  - Surgery for correction of a cleft lip and palate can result in scar tissue, which can make arch expansion difficult to achieve.

16.5.4 Habit

- A constant *digit sucking habit* can result in a crossbite.
  - A crossbite appears due to the duration and intensity of the habit, which can have an impact on the dental arch.
  - The posterior segment of the upper arch becomes narrow due to the pressure from the tongue and cheeks as the thumb/finger applies pressure anteriorly, which changes the archform, resulting in a crossbite.

16.6 Treatment of Crossbites

16.6.1 Interceptive (Early) Treatment

- *Thumb/digit dissuader*:
  - This procedure is used in patients with a digit sucking habit.
  - The digit dissuader is used to cease the habit.

- This is achieved by the dissuader feeling uncomfortable on the thumb/finger when the patient tries to continue this habit, which eventually results into ceasing the habit.
- It is mainly used on patients aged 7–8 years old, when the central incisors, lateral incisors and first permanent molars have erupted and the habit continues.
- The dissuader can be on a fixed or removable appliance (Figures 16.4 and 16.5).

- *Quadhelix:*
  - A quadhelix (Figure 16.6) is a fixed appliance that cannot be removed.
  - The appliance can be used for interceptive treatment for early correction of the dentition.
  - The appliance is used to correct a crossbite by expanding the upper arch.
  - The appliance is also used for a repaired cleft maxilla to expand the arch.
  - The appliance can be active or passive:
    - Active is when it is used to help expansion by being adjusted.
    - Passive is when it is used after active treatment to help aid retention of expansion.
  - A quadhelix can also contain a fixed digit deterrent, which will help to stop a digit sucking habit.

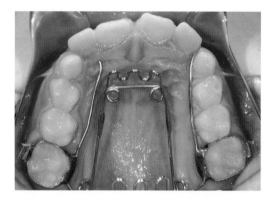

Figure 16.4 Fixed digit dissuader. Quadhelix incorporated with digit deterrent habit breaker.

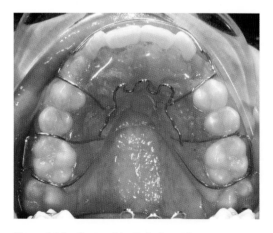

Figure 16.5 Removable digit dissuader.

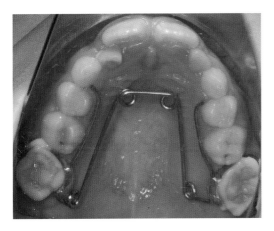

Figure 16.6 Quadhelix.

16.6.2 Removable Appliances

For correction of crossbites the following springs and screws can be incorporated within a removable appliance:
- Anterior expansion screw or Z springs (double cantilever):
  - Both of these active components will correct an anterior crossbite.
  - It is corrected by achieving labial movement of the anterior segment.
- Midline expansion screw or coffin spring:
  - Both of these active components will correct a posterior crossbite.
  - It is corrected by expanding the upper arch.
- 3D expansion screw:
  - This screw corrects both anterior and posterior crossbites.
  - This is achieved by expanding the upper arch to correct posterior crossbites and gaining labial movement of the anterior segment.
- All of these active components would be incorporated with posterior bite planes within the removable appliance. This is to open up the bite and dissuade any occlusal interference, which allows for the tooth/teeth to jump over the bite.

16.6.3 Functional Appliances

- *Frankel appliance*: this contains buccal shields to reduce the soft tissue pressures, which allows expansion of the arch passively.
- *Clark's twin block*: this can be modified by incorporating a midline expansion screw. As well as correcting the anterior/posterior arch relationship, it also corrects the transverse relationship due to the screw allowing for expansion.

16.6.4 Fixed Appliances

- *Anterior crossbite correction*:
  - Torque via rectangular archwires:
    - Torque can be applied to the teeth by the use of rectangular archwires.
    - This will help to upright the tooth/teeth out of an anterior crossbite.

- o When correcting an anterior crossbite, it is important to disarticulate the back teeth by incorporating a bite-disengaging technique. For example, placing posterior bite blocks will free any occlusal interference by opening the bite, allowing the tooth/teeth to jump the bite.
- *Posterior crossbite correction*:
  - Crossbite elastics:
    - o These can help to correct crossbites by bonding an attachment (buttons) onto the palatal surface of the upper tooth that is in crossbite.
    - o Elastics are then placed from the button to the bracket on the buccal surface of the lower dentition.
- Stainless-steel or titanium molybdenum alloy (TMA) archwires:
  - This type of archwire can be used to help with correction of a buccal crossbite.
  - Expanding the archwire before it is inserted into the bracket slots helps to expand the upper arch.
  - Archwires made of stainless steel or TMA are considered because once they have been adjusted and expanded, the archwire will be permanently set into its new formation, allowing correction to take place.
- *Lingual crossbite correction (scissorbite)*:
  - Lingual crossbite elastics:
    - o Elastics can help to correct a lingual crossbite.
    - o This is achieved by bonding an attachment (button) on the lingual surface of the lower tooth, with the elastic being run from the bonded attachment to the bracket on the buccal surface of the upper tooth.
  - Stainless-steel or TMA archwires:
    - o This type of archwire can be used to help with correction of a lingual crossbite.
    - o This is achieved by expanding the archwire before it is inserted into the bracket slot, which helps to expand the lower arch.
    - o Archwires made of stainless steel or TMA are considered because once they have been adjusted and expanded, the archwire will be permanently set in its new formation, allowing correction to take place.

16.6.5 Headgear

The facebow can be used to create expansion. Expansion is applied at the intermolar region, which expands the upper arch.

16.6.6 Surgery

- Rapid maxillary expansion (RME):
  - An RME (Figure 16.7) is a fixed appliance that cannot be removed by the patient and is used in the upper arch only.
  - It is used to achieve expansion of the upper arch, which will correct a posterior crossbite and gain expansion in a repaired cleft maxilla.
  - The appliance achieves skeletal expansion rather than dento-alveolar expansion.
  - The appliance contains a Hyrax screw, which is activated by the patient who turns the screw up to four times a day with a key while it is in the mouth. This produces up to 1 mm of movement a day.
  - Expansion is achieved by the appliance splitting the mid-palatine suture.
  - Once expansion is achieved, the appliance is left passively as a retainer for several (three) months. This prevents any relapse and allows for the bony infill of the expanded suture to take place.

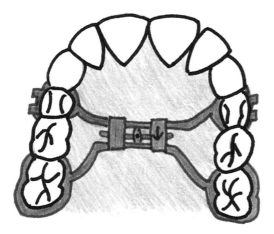

Figure 16.7 Rapid maxillary expansion.

16.7   Stability of a Crossbite

- Certain factors are important when ensuring the stability of a crossbite post-orthodontic treatment. The factors to consider are:
  - Ensuring a good stable overbite to prevent any anterior crossbites from relapsing.
  - A poor bite post-orthodontic treatment can result in relapse.
  - Once an anterior crossbite has been corrected, it is important to ensure the upper incisors cover one-third of the lower anterior incisors when the patient is in full occlusion. Failing to do so results in relapse by the anterior teeth moving back into crossbite due to no support from the lower incisors.
- Ensure the posterior teeth have not been tipped too much into the correct position.
  - If this is the case, the posterior teeth can relapse because the periodontal support around the teeth has been compromised.
- Good posterior occlusion.
  - Ensure the patient's posterior teeth are in good intercuspation, which will prevent any unwanted tooth movement.
  - Patients who do not have a full lock on the occlusion when biting together will relapse, enabling the posterior teeth to move palatally into a crossbite.
- Favourable antero-posterior and transverse skeletal growth.
  - To prevent relapse it is good to ensure that the patient has good antero-posterior and transverse skeletal growth.
  - Once a crossbite is corrected, if the patient still has skeletal growth they can relapse.

17

Centreline

The centreline is also known as the midline and is found between the upper and lower central incisors. Patients can present with a perfect centreline, with the upper and lower incisors matching. In some cases patients could present with a centreline discrepancy, with either or both off to the right- or left-hand side.

The idea is to have the upper centreline in line with the mid-facial plane when the patient smiles. The mid-facial plane runs vertically through the middle of the face between the eyes, down the nose, and right down the middle of the chin point. The lower midline should then be in line with the upper midline. However, this is not always the case and some patients present with the midline off to one side (Figure 17.1), which can be due to a number of reasons such as extractions, missing teeth, and supernumerary teeth.

However, there are many ways in which a centreline can be corrected.

17.1 Treatment Options

17.1.1 Removable Appliance

- This would be considered with patients who are in the early mixed dentition.
- Centreline correction would be achieved by tipping with palatal springs and a unilateral extraction.

17.1.2 Functional Appliance

- If there is a lower centreline shift and the patient is going into a functional appliance, the wax bite can help correct the centrelines.
- This is achieved by making the upper and lower centrelines coincide with each other when taking the wax bite, but this can only be done if there is a lower centreline shift.

17.1.3 Fixed Appliances

To correct a centreline with fixed appliances, the following techniques/procedures can be used:

- Extractions of the first premolar on one side and the second premolar on the other, for example the first premolar taken on the side you want to move round to.
- Laceback on one side (the side that you want to shift round) to distalise the canine.

Textbook for Orthodontic Therapists, First Edition. Ceri Davies.
© 2020 John Wiley & Sons Ltd. Published 2020 by John Wiley & Sons Ltd.

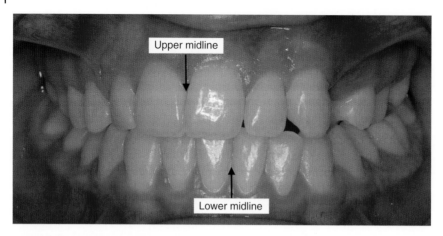

Figure 17.1 Centric view of an upper midline shift.

- Chain elastic to move one tooth at a time round.
- Push pull mechanics: a coil spring to help push the midline over, and a chain to also help guide the midline round.
- Midline intermaxillary elastics – class II on the side you want to move round, class III on the other side.

17.1.4 Surgery

The following surgical procedures can be considered:

- Distraction osteogenesis:
  - Considered in patients with a severe skeletal deformity.
  - Reconstruction will help to repair the deformity and correct the midline.
- Bilateral sagittal split osteotomy (BSSO):
  - Considered in patients with a severe skeletal deformity.
  - Maxilla and mandible are cut and moved to match up with one another, allowing the centrelines to coincide.

18

Overjets

An overjet is the distance between the upper and lower incisors in the horizontal plane (Figure 18.1). A normal overjet is 2–4 mm, whereas an increased overjet is anything over 5 mm (Figure 18.2).

18.1 Treatment Options

18.1.1 Removable Appliance

The following active components can be used to help retract the upper incisors:

- Roberts retractor
- Active labial bow.

Activation is achieved by squeezing the U loops together, which activates the bow to retract the incisors. The orthodontist can only do activation of active components.

18.1.2 Functional Appliance

The functional appliance used to help retract an overjet is a Clark's twin block. This helps to posture the lower mandible forward, achieving reduction of the upper anterior segment.

18.1.3 Fixed Appliance

The following techniques/procedures can be considered to help reduce an overjet, but only in a working stainless-steel archwire:

- Power chain:
  - This may be considered in patients who are not good with their elastics and treatment is being compromised.
- Retraction nickel titanium (NiTi) closing coils (intra-arch mechanics):
  - The patient has had extraction of U4s.
  - U5–U7s have been undertied to prevent forward movement.
  - Retraction NiTi closing coils are used to retract back the anterior segment.

Textbook for Orthodontic Therapists, First Edition. Ceri Davies.
© 2020 John Wiley & Sons Ltd. Published 2020 by John Wiley & Sons Ltd.

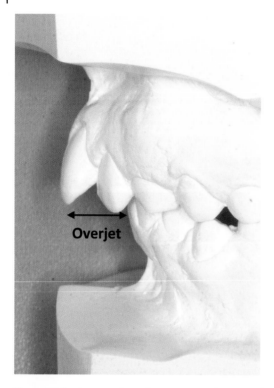

Figure 18.1 Increased overjet on pre-treatment study model.

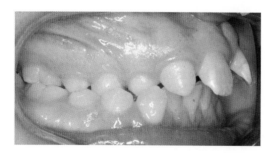

Figure 18.2 Right buccal intra-oral photograph of an increased overjet.

- Intra-arch elastics – class I:
  - U5–U7s have been undertied to prevent forward movement.
  - Class I elastic placed from U3s to U7s to help retract the overjet.
- Inter-arch elastics – class II:
  - Class II elastics used from U3s to L6s/L7s.
  - This allows retraction of the upper anterior segment and proclination of the lower anterior segment to reduce the overjet.
- Round archwires
  - These are used to roll back the incisors.
  - No torque is achieved, but the root apex remains in the opposite direction to the crown.

18.1.4 Surgery

- Bilateral Sagittal Split Osteotomy (BSSO):
    - Considered in severe cases.
    - Used for mandibular advancement to reduce the overjet.
- Le Fort I
    - Incisions made to free the maxilla.
    - Considered to advance the maxilla to reduce the overjet.

19

Bimaxillary Proclination

19.1   Definition

Bimaxillary proclination is a term used to describe occlusions where both the upper and lower incisors are proclined (Figure 19.1). It is more commonly seen in some racial groups (for example African Caribbean).

19.2   Aetiology

Bimaxillary proclination can be due to the following:

- Weak muscular tone, where there is no support to control the dentition, allowing the incisors to procline.
- Forward tongue position or macroglossia tongue. Due to the position and size of the tongue, the incisors can be proclined.
- Inclination of incisors.

19.3   Relapse

The reason for relapse after treatment can be due to the following:

- Forward tongue position or macroglossia tongue.
- Spaces occurring distal to the 3s.

19.4   Retention

Means of retention when retaining a bimaxillary proclination case:

- Bonded retainer 4–4
- Vacuum form retainers
- Wrap-around Hawley – use of labial bow to control incisors.

Textbook for Orthodontic Therapists, First Edition. Ceri Davies.
© 2020 John Wiley & Sons Ltd. Published 2020 by John Wiley & Sons Ltd.

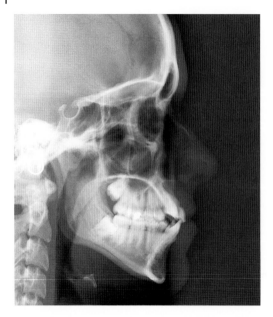

Figure 19.1 Cephalometric radiograph. Bimaxillary proclination of upper and lower incisors.

20

Growth Rotations

Growth rotations occur as a result of different amounts of growth of the posterior and anterior face heights. There are two types of growth rotation:

- Forward growth rotation (Figure 20.1). Features of this are:
  - Decreased lower face height
  - Class II malocclusion
  - Deepbite
  - Increased overbite.
- Backward growth rotation (Figure 20.2). Features of this are:
  - Increased lower face height
  - Class III malocclusion
  - Anterior overbite
  - Decreased overbite.

The more common growth rotation is forward growth rotation.

Figure 20.1 Forward growth rotation.

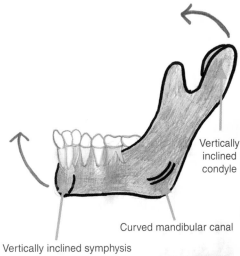

Vertically inclined condyle

Curved mandibular canal

Vertically inclined symphysis

Textbook for Orthodontic Therapists, First Edition. Ceri Davies.
© 2020 John Wiley & Sons Ltd. Published 2020 by John Wiley & Sons Ltd.

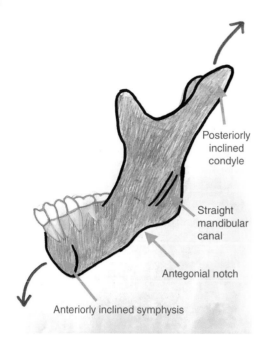

Figure 20.2 Backward growth rotation.

21

Tooth Movement

21.1 Biomechanics of Tooth Movement

21.1.1 Centre of Resistance

The centre of resistance is the point in the body where the resistance to movement is concentrated. When moving a tooth, the force that is applied must hit its centre of resistance to enable it to move.

For example:

- For bodily movement to occur to an object, the force must be directly applied to its centre of resistance.

In orthodontics:

- For a tooth to move, the force cannot be directly applied to the centre of resistance. This is because the centre of resistance on a tooth does not coincide with the centre of mass.
- All three planes of space should be visualised with the centre of resistance of a tooth.

Where is the centre of rotation found?

- For *single-rooted teeth*, the centre of resistance is found approximately halfway down the root surface.
- For *multi-rooted teeth*, the centre of resistance is found in the area of the root furcation (Figure 21.1).
- *Furcation* is the area found at the dip of the root on multi-rooted teeth for the centre of resistance. If the alveolar bone and gingiva recede away, the centre of resistance will move apically. This is found in patients who present with bone loss and recession.
- *Maxilla:* the centre of resistance on the maxilla is found in the premolar region. With high pull headgear, maxillary restraint is achieved. This is because the pull of the headgear goes through the centre of resistance.
- *Mandible:* the centre of resistance on the mandible is by the lower premolars around the angle of the mandible.

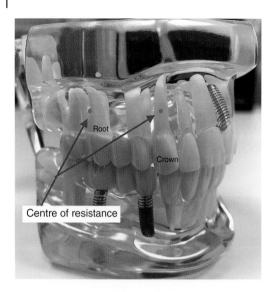

Figure 21.1 Centre of resistance on single- and multi-rooted teeth.

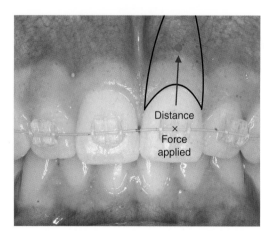

Figure 21.2 Force moment at one point of force. A central view of aesthetic fixed appliances on the upper arch. The direction of the UR1 root is drawn, showing the centre of resistance halfway up. The force applied to the tooth by engagement of the archwire and bracket is multiplied by the distance between where the force is applied and the centre of resistance.

21.1.2 Force Moment

A force moment (Figure 21.2) helps to describe a type of force that is created which causes rotational movement. The moment of a force is the component found within the force. This component will cause *rotational movement only*.

A force moment is described as:

> Magnitude of force applied to tooth × Perpendicular distance between point of application and centre of resistance

The whole process equals the moment. This achieves *rotational movement only*, but there can be tipping too. *Tipping* is achieved when the line of force that is created does not pass through the centre of resistance. Due to this, the force will translate and rotate the tooth around its centre of resistance.

For example, a palatally displaced lateral incisor with a button bonded on the labial surface of the incisor with chain elastic engaged from the button to the archwire will help bring the tooth anteriorly.

21.1.3 Force Couple

In fixed appliances, when an archwire connects into a bracket slot a force couple is created (Figure 21.3). A force couple will achieve the following movements:

- Rotation
- Inclination of teeth
- Torque.

Two equal and opposite forces produce a force couple which acts to cause rotation. The size of the couple is described as:

Magnitude of forces applied to tooth × Distance between them

All together this equals a force couple, which achieves pure rotation around the tooth's centre of resistance. No translation is achieved. For example, a force couple is achieved when an archwire is engaged into the bracket slot.

21.1.4 Force Couple and Moment

However, force moments and force couples do work together. By them working together this will produce bodily movement (Figure 21.4).

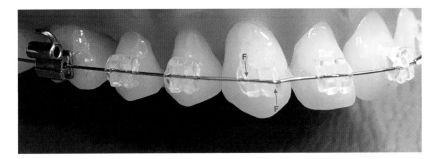

Figure 21.3 Force couple. Aesthetic ice brackets showing full engagement of an archwire with elastomeric modules. UR3 shows two points of equal and opposite forces from full engagement of the archwire.

Figure 21.4 Force couple and moment. Bodily movement being achieved on a lower incisor by a force couple and moment working together. When the archwire is engaged into the bracket slot, the force couple created is used to control the tipping that is caused by the force moment. This achieves bodily tooth movement, for example when the archwire is engaged into the bracket slot (couple) and chain elastic is placed 6-6 to help bring the teeth back.

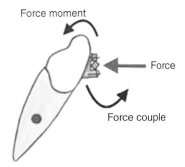

Force moment

Force

Force couple

21.2 Types of Tooth Movement

There are six different types of tooth movement that can be produced:

- Tipping
- Bodily movement
- Torque
- Rotation
- Extrusion
- Intrusion.

21.2.1 Tipping

- This tooth movement produces 30–60 g of force.
- Tipping occurs when in one given direction of force the clinical crown moves more than its root (Figure 21.5).
- This is seen when the tooth tips around its centre of resistance, with the crown and root moving in the opposite direction to each other.

21.2.2 Bodily Movement

- This tooth movement produces 60–120 g of force.
- Bodily movement occurs when both the crown and the root move an equal distance in the same direction (Figure 21.6).

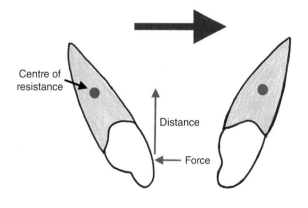

Figure 21.5 Tipping movement being achieved.

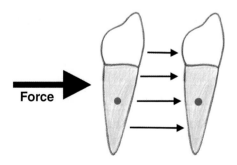

Figure 21.6 Bodily movement being achieved.

21.2.3 Torque

- This tooth movement produces 50–100 g of force.
- Torque achieves movement of the root in a bucco-lingual direction with minimal or no crown movement (Figure 21.7).
- This is seen when the crown and the root are in the opposite direction, for example the crown may be labially inclined, but the root may be lying back palatally.

21.2.4 Rotation

- This tooth movement produces 30–60 g of force.
- Rotation occurs when a mesial or distal force is applied to the labial/buccal surface of a tooth to help achieve rotation (Figure 21.8).

Figure 21.7   Torque being achieved.

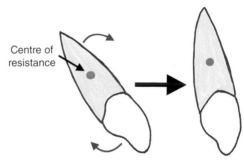

Centre of resistance

Rectangular wire angulated into bracket slot to achieve root torque

Figure 21.8   Rotational movement (of UL3) being achieved.

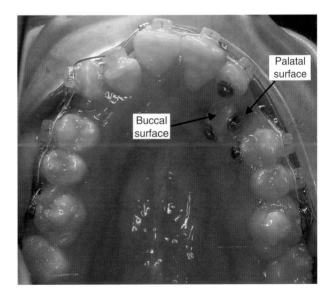

Palatal surface

Buccal surface

21.2.5 Extrusion

- This tooth movement produces 30–60 g of force.
- Extrusion occurs when the tooth itself is moved out of its socket (Figure 21.9), causing stretching of its periodontal ligament (PDL).

21.2.6 Intrusion

- This tooth movement produces 10–20 g of force.
- Intrusion occurs when the tooth itself is moved into its socket (Figure 21.10), causing compression of its PDL.

21.3 Biology of Tooth Movement

21.3.1 Facts of Tooth Movement

- Gentle forces that are constantly applied to a tooth for a period of time will make the tooth move.
- Applying continuous force to a tooth results in:
  - Remodelling of the alveolar bone
  - Reorganisation of the PDL
  - Changes in the periodontium.

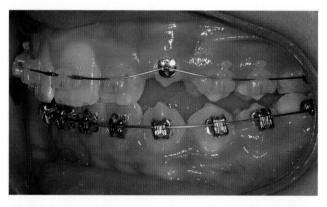

Figure 21.9 Extrusion movement (of UL3) being achieved.

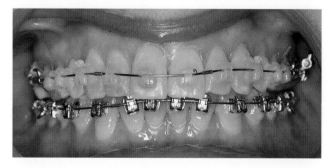

Figure 21.10 Intrusion movement (of UR1) being achieved, with the bracket positioned more incisally.

- The PDL is made up of:
  - Cells, blood vessels, collagen fibres
  - Alveolar bone
  - Cementum.
- Alveolar bone is capable of:
  - Remodelling
  - Repair
  - Regeneration.

21.3.2 Forces Applied to a Tooth

- There are two types of forces that can be applied to a tooth (Tables 21.1 and 21.2):
  - Optimum force
  - Excessive force.
- A preferred force of 20–26 g/cm^3 is ideal to move a tooth by a continual force that is acting for more than six hours a day.

21.3.3 Pressure/Tension Theory

When a force is applied to a tooth, it results in areas of compression (pressure) and tension within the PDL. Bone is resorbed on the compression side and bone is deposited on the tension side. This is the pressure/tension theory (Figure 21.11).

Table 21.1 Histology of a light force.

---

1. **Optimum force is applied to the tooth – light force**
   Does not occlude capillary pressure – blood is flowable

2. **Chemical messengers trigger cellular reactions**
   Chemicals: prostaglandins, cytokines, and nitric oxide

3. **Results in area of pressure and tension**

4. **Cells react to force**
   Osteoblasts:
   - Found on tension side – 48 hours after force is applied
   - Deposit bone
   - Cells are stretched and flattened
   - Recruit and activate osteoclasts

   Osteoclasts:
   - Found on pressure side – 48 hours after force is applied
   - Resorb bone in front of the root

   Osteocytes:
   - Used to be osteoblasts, turn to osteocytes in mineralised bone
   - Detect mechanical load on the bone

5. **Alveolar bone changes**
   Allow physiological tooth movement (good)
   Result in frontal resorption

Table 21.2 Histology of an excessive force.

1. **Excessive force is applied to the tooth – heavy force**
   Occludes capillary pressure – blood is not flowable = cells die
2. **Chemical messengers trigger cellular reactions**
   Chemicals: prostaglandins, cytokines, and nitric oxide
3. **Results in area of pressure and tension**
4. **Sterile necrosis appears in periodontal ligament – cell death**
   Results in hyalinization due to capillaries being occluded
5. **Cells react to force**
   Osteoblasts:
   - Found on tension side – 48 hours after force is applied
   - Deposit bone
   - Cells are stretched and flattened more
   - Recruit and activate osteoclasts
   Osteoclasts:
   - Found on pressure side – 48 hours after force is applied
   - Resorb bone beneath area of necrosis adjacent to hyalinisation within a few days after force is applied
   Osteocytes:
   - Used to be osteoblasts, turn to osteocytes in mineralised bone
   - Detect mechanical load on the bone
6. **Tooth movement is delayed by 7–14 days**
7. **Alveolar bone changes**
   Allow pathological tooth movement (bad)
   Result in undermining resorption

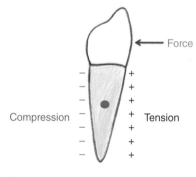

Figure 21.11 Pressure/tension theory.

21.3.4 Cellular Responses

There are many cells that are involved in the cellular response, such as:

- Osteoblasts
- Osteoclasts
- Osteocytes
- Fibroblasts
- Cementoclasts
- Cementoblasts.

Within a few hours of the force being applied to the tooth, the cellular response is seen. Once the force has been applied to the tooth, the following chemicals are detected in the PDL:

- Prostaglandin
- Cytokines
- Nitric oxide.

These chemicals cause the release of cells involved in the cellular response (osteoblasts, osteo-clasts, osteocytes).

- *Osteoblasts* are found on the tension side, 48 hours after a force has been applied.
  - They deposit bone.
  - They are the control cells as they recruit and activate the osteoclasts.
  - They become osteocytes when surrounded by mineralised bone.

  They have four main functions:
  - They produce bone and matrix.
  - They recruit and activate osteoclasts.
  - They are the main regulators of bone.
  - They send messages to inhibit osteoclasts to tell them to stop working.
- *Osteoclasts* are found on the compression (pressure) side, 48 hours after a force has been applied.
  - They are large cells known as multinucleate cells, which are the main cells that are involved in bone resorption.
  - Resorption occurs more rapidly than deposition.
  - They are under the control of osteoblasts.
- *Osteocytes* are responsible for detecting mechanical load (force) on the bone. They used to be osteoblasts, but turn to osteocytes when surrounded by mineralised bone.
- *Fibroblasts* are cells that help in remodelling of the PDL. They are part of the resorption of exist-ing fibres and formation of new fibres. They produce and destroy collagen fibres.
- *Cementoclasts* resorb the necrotic tissue and also the root surface (cementum). These cells occur in undermining resorption due to excessive forces being applied.
- *Cementoblasts* are cells that take part in the formation of the cementum. They deposit bone around the cementum.

21.3.5 Resorption

There are two types of resorption (Figure 21.12):

- *Frontal resorption*, which occurs when an optimum force is applied to a tooth. Bone is resorbed in front of the root on the compressed area.
- *Undermining resorption*, which occurs when an excessive force is applied to a tooth. Bone is resorbed from beneath the area of necrosis adjacent to the hyalinized area, which is the area which appears translucent when viewed under a microscope.

Clinical signs of frontal resorption:

- No complaint from the patient of any prolonged discomfort.
- Movement of the teeth is happening gradually.
- No excessive mobility found among the teeth.

Clinical signs of undermining resorption:

- Complaining from patient of prolonged discomfort.
- Mobility is found among the teeth.
- Tooth movement is delayed, or tooth does not move and then suddenly jumps.
- Root resorption occurs.
- No signs can be seen at all.

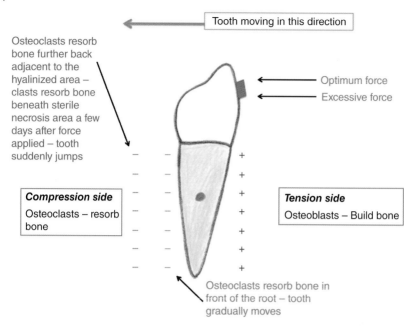

Tooth moving in this direction

Osteoclasts resorb bone further back adjacent to the hyalinized area – clasts resorb bone beneath sterile necrosis area a few days after force applied – tooth suddenly jumps

Optimum force

Excessive force

Compression side

Osteoclasts – resorb bone

Tension side

Osteoblasts – Build bone

Osteoclasts resorb bone in front of the root – tooth gradually moves

Figure 21.12   Different levels of force on a tooth.

21.3.6   Factors to Consider for Rate of Tooth Movement

- Light ideal forces are applied to teeth 24 hours a day.
- Continuous force is applied for at least 6 hours a day.
- A tooth movement rate of 1 mm a month is achieved.
- Every individual responds to treatment differently, so some are quicker and some slower than others. This is dependent on the response of the cellular reaction and the density of their alveolar bone.
- Adult treatment is known to be slower due to the reduced cellularity and vascularity and density of their alveolar bone.

21.3.7   Compression and Tension Areas for Individual Tooth Movements

Figures 21.13–21.18 illustrate the areas of compression and tension for the various kinds of tooth movements.

Figure 21.13 Area of compression and tension for bodily movement. Bodily movement of UR7 moving mesial into the UR6 place. An even compressive load is being resorbed mesial to UR7 to allow for bodily movement of UR7 to close the space between UR7 and UR5 due to the missing UR6. While bone is being resorbed mesially, regeneration of bone occurs on the distal side of UR7. PDL, periodontal ligament.

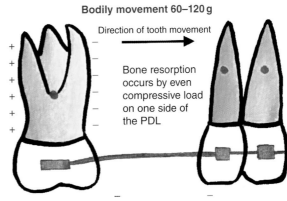

Bodily movement 60–120 g

Direction of tooth movement

Bone resorption occurs by even compressive load on one side of the PDL

(Tension side)   (Compressed side)
Regenerating bone   Resorbing bone
osteoblasts found   osteoclasts found

Figure 21.14 Area of compression and tension for tipping movement. Resorbing and regenerating bone to allow tipping movement of UR1. Study models presenting with class II div II incisors with drawn root for UR1. To allow for proclination of the upper central incisors, bone is diagonally resorbed by the alveolar crest and root apex at opposite ends, allowing for proclination of the UR1. Bone is then regenerated also in the opposite sides of the root from the resorption at the alveolar crest and root apex. PDL, periodontal ligament.

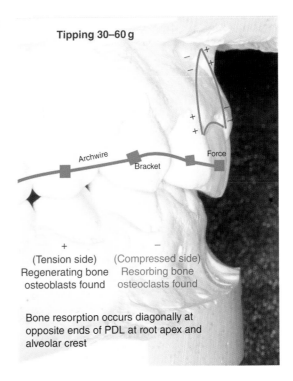

Tipping 30–60 g

Archwire   Force
Bracket

(Tension side)   (Compressed side)
Regenerating bone   Resorbing bone
osteoblasts found   osteoclasts found

Bone resorption occurs diagonally at opposite ends of PDL at root apex and alveolar crest

Figure 21.15 Area of compression and tension for extrusion movement. Bone resorption occurs at the alveolar crest as the tooth is being extruded out of the socket.

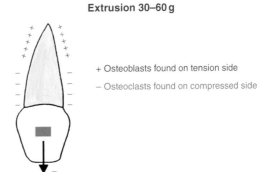

Extrusion 30–60 g

+ Osteoblasts found on tension side
− Osteoclasts found on compressed side

Force

Intrusion 10–20 g

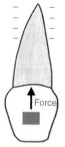

+ Osteoblasts found on tension side

− Osteoclasts found on compressed side

Force

Figure 21.16 Area of compression for intrusion movement. Bone resorption occurs at the root apex.

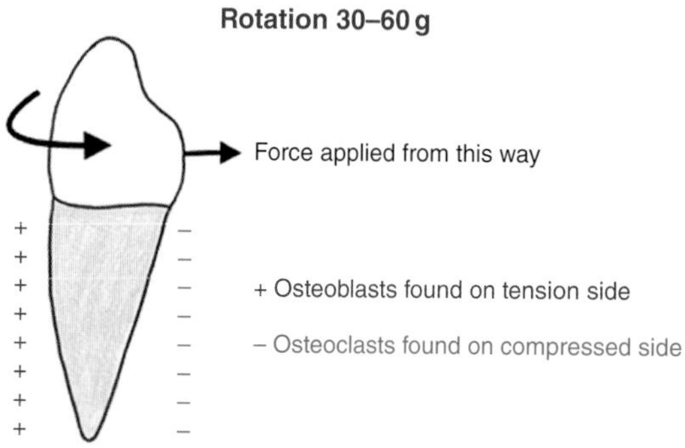

Rotation 30–60 g

Force applied from this way

+ Osteoblasts found on tension side

− Osteoclasts found on compressed side

Figure 21.17 Area of compression and tension for rotational movement. Bone resorption occurs on the even compressed side on which the tooth is being rotated.

Torque 50–100 g

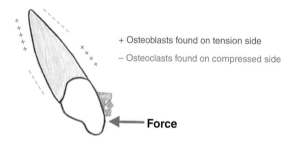

+ Osteoblasts found on tension side

− Osteoclasts found on compressed side

Force

Figure 21.18 Area of compression and tension for torque movement. Bone resorption occurs diagonally at the opposite ends of the periodontal ligament at the root apex and alveolar crest.

22

Impressions

Impressions are a negative reproduction of the dental structures. Impressions are frequently used and are taken for many reasons in orthodontics:

- Study models:
  This is for a record of the patient's teeth.
  - All patients will have a set of impressions taken pre- and post-orthodontic treatment. These are then stored away for records showing the teeth at the initial stage and the final stage.
  - These study models are also used for Peer Assessment Rating (PAR) scoring in the UK National Health Service (NHS), which measures the success of treatment for each individual patient (see Chapter 34).
- Making an appliance such as an upper removable appliance or functional appliance:
  - Impressions are also taken when making an appliance for the patient.
  - Some patients may have a removable appliance or functional appliance as their first stage of treatment before fixed appliances.
  - The impressions are taken and then sent off to the lab, which will cast the impressions up and then make the appliance.
- Vacuum formed retainers:
  - Impressions are taken to enable the production of vacuum formed retainers.
  - These impressions are casted up into study models and the retainers are then made from them.
  - Some orthodontic practices may send their impressions off to a lab for the retainers to be made, and some have their own in-house lab at the practice.

22.1   Materials Used for Impression Taking

Impressions can be taken out of two types of materials:

- Alginate
- Poly-vinyl siloxane (PVS), a silicone material.

Textbook for Orthodontic Therapists, First Edition. Ceri Davies.
© 2020 John Wiley & Sons Ltd. Published 2020 by John Wiley & Sons Ltd.

22.1.1   Constituents of Alginate

The following ingredients are found in alginate:

- Sodium alginate
- Calcium sulphate
- Tri-sodium phosphate, which slows the setting time
- Glycols, to make it dustless
- Flavours and colouring.

22.1.2   Advantages and Disadvantages of Alginate

Advantages:

- Easy to use.
- Material can provide good surface detail.
- Material can provide good compatibility with oral tissues.
- Material is low cost.
- Some materials can come with a pleasant taste.
- It has a rapid set time.
- It is relatively firm.

   Disadvantages:

- Material can tear easily.
- Provides poor dimensional stability.
- Poor adhesion to the tray can result in material not sticking.
- Material is difficult to disinfect.
- Impression can distort more quickly due to the material drying out.

22.1.3   PVS

PVS comes in liquid form and has two separate components, which once mixed together cure and harden very quickly. PVS use is very popular for manufacturing Invisalign appliances (see Chapter 40) because of the good surface detail the material gives.

   Advantages:

- Can provide good surface detail.
- Less risk of distortion.
- Can be well tolerated by patients.
- Impression can be duplicated, which is good for Kesling models (see Chapter 10).

   Disadvantages:

- Harder to use.
- Increase in cost.
- Longer working time.
- Requires good technique.

22.1.4 Ideal Impression Material

There are eight properties to consider when you want the ideal impression material to help manufacture plaster models:

- Accuracy
- Flexibility – non-tearing
- Short setting time
- Ease of mixing
- Biocompatibility
- Ease of disinfection
- Long shelf life
- Pleasant taste
- Cost efficiency

22.2 Technique for Taking an Impression

1) Make sure the patient is sitting up – a patient lying down while impressions are taken may want to gag due to the impression material running down the back of their throat.
2) Ensure the patient is relaxed, which is achieved by good communication.
3) Select the appropriate size of tray with/without adhesive – it is always good to try different sizes before mixing the material. If a tray is inserted into the mouth loaded with alginate and is too small, it is more than likely that a mess will be created where the material is not set.
4) Make the appropriate mix – ensure a good smooth mix of the alginate with no air bubbles (Figure 22.1).
5) Load the tray with alginate with the use of a spatula, ensuring it is evenly spread out.
6) Seat the impression in the mouth, ensuring that the teeth and gums do not touch the side of the tray.
7) Ensure the midline is correct to the tray – line the midline up with the handle of the tray.
8) Remove the tray gently to break the vacuum seal.
9) Check the impression to ensure all aspects of the gums and teeth are present (Figures 22.2 and 22.3).

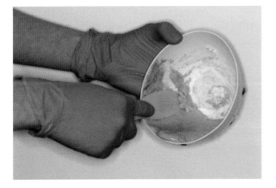

Figure 22.1 Alginate mixing.

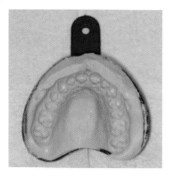

Figure 22.2 Upper impression.

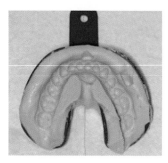

Figure 22.3 Lower impression.

10) Disinfect the impression by placing it in hydrochloride for 10 minutes (see next section).
11) Send the impression to the lab, ensuring it is fully wrapped in cold paper towels to ensure it keeps moist and does not dry out.

22.3 Technique for Disinfecting an Impression

1) Rinse the impression under cold water.
2) Immerse it in hydrochloride 0.1% for 10 minutes.
3) Rinse, bag, and label the impression and keep it moist by wrapping it in a cold paper towel. Failing to do this results in the impression drying out and becoming distorted, making it unusable.

23

Study Models

Study models are a positive reproduction of the dental structures. They have great importance within orthodontic treatment and are created for a record of pre- and post-treatment. As well as being part of a record, they are also used to help make retainers, removable appliances, and functional appliances, and to achieve a Peer Assessment Rating (PAR) score within the NHS.

Pre- and post-treatment study models are a minimum requirement for each individual patient.

23.1 Production of Study Models

Gypsum products, otherwise known as stone and plaster, make study models, and are mixed together to form a plaster material. Plaster is used because it is softer and more porous and can be polished.

The plaster is placed into the impression to produce the study models. Once the plaster has been poured into the impression, it is left to set and dry before it is removed.

23.2 What Are Study Models Used For?

- Diagnosis:
  - Study models are used to help with a treatment plan.
  - They help to look at the best course of treatment for each individual patient.
- Measurement – PAR, space analysis:
  - Study models are used to help gain measurements.
  - Space analysis using study models helps to determine how much crowding the patient has and how much space needs to be created (see Chapter 35).
  - PAR is used in the NHS to measure the success of treatment. Measurements are taken from pre- and post-study models to determine the overall success of treatment (see Chapter 34).
- Assessment of progress
- Illustration
- Medico-legal reasons:
  - As part of a legal requirement to make up the patient record.
- Education

Textbook for Orthodontic Therapists, First Edition. Ceri Davies.
© 2020 John Wiley & Sons Ltd. Published 2020 by John Wiley & Sons Ltd.

23.3 Technique for Production of Study Models

1) The first stage is the impression, which is a negative reproduction which is then disinfected in hydrochloride for 10 minutes and taken to the lab (see Chapter 22).
2) Gypsum (a plaster/stone product) is needed to help cast up the study model from the impression. This is water and powder mixed together at a ratio of 1 : 2.
3) The plaster must be mixed to a creamy, thick consistency to minimise any air bubbles.
4) The plaster is then poured into the impression, with a gentle flow of plaster into the occlusal and incisal surfaces.
5) Once poured, a base is then made for the study models, which can either be done by hand or a template. The base is important, as it ensures that when the study models are together, they are in the patient's natural occlusion when held up (Figures 23.1 and 23.2).

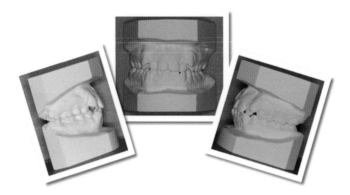

Figure 23.1 Centric, right buccal, and left buccal views of study models.

Figure 23.2 Upper and lower occlusal views of study models.

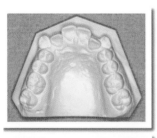

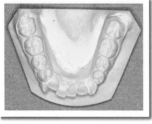

24

Radiographs

A radiograph is an image produced on a film by an X-ray. Radiographs can be developed either manually or digitally.

24.1   When Are Radiographs Taken?

Radiographs are only taken:

- After clinical examination of the patient.
- When clinically justified.

24.2   Types of Radiographs

- Dental panoramic tomography (DPT)
- Cephalometric (ceph) X-ray (see Chapter 25)
- Upper standard occlusal (USO)
- Periapical (PA)
- 3D cone beam computed tomography (CBCT) scan.

24.3   Why Do We Take Radiographs?

Radiographs are taken to help aid diagnosis and treatment planning.
    When recording the findings, the acronym PPP should be used, which stands for:

P – Presence
P – Position
P – Pathology

P – Presence:

- This looks at the presence of the teeth.
- It records any missing teeth (hypodontia) and extra teeth (supernumeraries).

Textbook for Orthodontic Therapists, First Edition. Ceri Davies.
© 2020 John Wiley & Sons Ltd. Published 2020 by John Wiley & Sons Ltd.

P – Position:

- This looks at the position and degree of development of the dentition.
- It records any unerupted teeth, impacted teeth, or ectopic teeth.

P – Pathology:

- This looks at any disease/infection that is found, such as:
  - Oral health (OH), caries, decay, gum disease, fractured root, root resorption, cysts, ankylosis, abscesses, access degree of restorations, root morphology, apical pathology
- Pathology studies pathogens, microbes which can cause disease.

24.4 Panoramic Radiographs

24.4.1 What Is a DPT?

A DPT is a radiograph that gives a two-dimensional view of the upper and lower jaws (maxilla and mandible).

24.4.2 Why Do We Take a DPT?

A DPT is taken to look at PPP: presence, position, and pathology, and is a general scan of the whole dentition.

24.4.3 How Does a DPT Help Us?

A DPT will help to look at:

- *Presence*: a DPT will look at any missing teeth or extra teeth such as hypodontia and supernumeraries.
- *Position*: a DPT will help look at the position and degree of the developing dentition:
  - Unerupted teeth
  - Impacted teeth caused by any obstruction such as crowding
  - Ectopic teeth
  - Transposition, seen on the canines, first premolars, and lower incisors
  - Ankylosis, seen on the first and second deciduous molars
  - Crowding.
- *Pathology*: This will help to locate any disease/infection that could be present. The DPT can help identify any:
  - Caries – due to poor OH
  - Decay – due to poor OH
  - Abscess
  - Gum disease
  - Fractured root
  - Root resorption
  - Cysts
  - Ankylosed teeth.

A DPT is not always a good X-ray to take when assessing bad OH. If a patient presents with bad OH, they should be referred back to their general dental practitioner for bitewings and periapicals to look for any interproximal caries.

24.4.4 When Do We Take a DPT?

A DPT is taken after a clinical examination and when clinically justified.

24.4.5 Locating the Position of Impacted Canines on a DPT

A special technique can be used to locate a position of an impacted canine; however, this should be done with care. To be 100% sure of the position, the parallax technique should be employed:

- If the canine presents bigger than its opposing canine, it means it is positioned palatally.
  - This is because it is in the focal trough, making it magnified.
- If the canine presents small compared to its opposing canine, it means it is positioned buccally.
  - This is because it is not in the focal trough.

When assessing this, always compare the impacted canine to the other canine. If the canines are both impacted, the position cannot be assessed and parallax is needed to be sure of their position.

24.5 Upper Standard Occlusal (USO)

24.5.1 What Is a USO?

A USO radiograph is a radiograph of the anterior part of the maxilla and anterior teeth.

24.5.2 Why Do We Take a USO?

A USO radiograph looks at PPP: presence, position, and pathology. It is often used to give a clearer reading of something that may be seen on a DPT in the midline.

24.5.3 How Does a USO Help Us?

A USO radiograph will help us look at:

- *Presence*: this will help to look at the presence of unerupted teeth such as canines and any supernumeraries like mesiodens.
- *Position*: the parallax technique is used and helps us to locate the position of unerupted canines.
  - There are two types of parallax that can be used:
    - Horizontal
    - Vertical.
  - With a USO radiograph the vertical parallax is used, which involves the use of DPT too.
  - First, a DPT is taken which looks at the position of the canine, followed by a USO radiograph
  - These two X-rays they are then compared using the acronym SLOB (Same, Lingual, Opposite, Buccal) to help locate the position of the unerupted canine.
    - If the canine/tooth moves in the same direction as the tube head on the X-ray, then the tooth is positioned in a lingual or palatal position.
    - If the canine/tooth moves in the opposite direction to the tube head, then the tooth is in a buccal position.
  - Even though the technique is used to locate the position of a tooth, it is also used when an exposure is needed, as it is important for the surgeon to know the correct position during surgery when exposing a tooth.

- *Pathology*: this area will help to locate any disease/infection such as:
  - Caries – due to poor OH
  - Decay – due to poor OH
  - Abscess
  - Gum disease
  - Fractured root
  - Root resorption
  - Cysts
  - Ankylosed teeth
  - Root morphology
  - Root resorption
  - Apical pathology

24.5.4   When Do We Take a USO?

Only when clinically justified after clinical examination of the patient.

24.6   Parallax Technique

Parallax is a technique that is used when assessing or localising the position of an unerupted tooth/teeth.

This is most commonly when a tooth needs to be located for an exposure, so its position can be identified for the surgeon and clinicians can pull the tooth in the correct direction.

There are two types of parallax:

- Horizontal
- Vertical.

Parallax works by taking two radiographic views of the unerupted tooth with the tube head in two different positions. Assessing the direction in which the tooth has moved from both radiographs identifies the position of the unerupted tooth.

24.6.1   Assessing the Position of the Canine

To locate the position of an impacted canine, the acronym SLOB is used:

S – Same
L – Lingual/palatal
O – Opposite
B – Buccal

- *Lingual/palatal positioned canines*: if the tooth moves in the same direction as the tube head of the X-ray, then the tooth is positioned in a lingual or palatal position.
- *Buccal positioned canines*: if the tooth moves in the opposite direction to the tube head, then the tooth is in a buccal position.

24.6.2 Horizontal Parallax

Radiographs used for horizontal parallax consist of two PAs or two PAs and a USO radiograph.

This type of parallax moves the tube head around the arch in the horizontal plane for each radiographic image (left to right).

24.6.3 Vertical Parallax

Radiographs used for vertical parallax consist of a DPT and a USO radiograph.

This type of parallax moves the tube head in the vertical plane, which changes the degree of angulation between the two radiographic images.

- DPT: tube head is aimed upwards at 8°.
- USO: tube head is aimed downwards at 65°.

24.7 Periapical Radiographs

A periapical (PA) radiograph can be used to assess the presence, position and pathology of any unerupted teeth.

- *Position*: the parallax technique can be used with a periapical radiograph. Horizontal parallax involves the use of 2 PAs or 2 PAs and an USO radiograph. This technique will help to locate the position of an impacted canine.
- *Pathology*: a PA radiograph can also help to assess pathology, such as:
  - Caries – due to poor oral health (OH)
  - Decay – due to poor OH
  - Abscess
  - Gum disease
  - Fractured root
  - Root resorption
  - Cysts
  - Ankylosed teeth
  - Root morphology
  - Root resorption
  - Apical pathology

24.8 Reasons for Taking Radiographs

There are many reasons for taking radiographs, which must be considered prior to taking the image:

- To assess abnormalities:
  - Size
  - Shape
  - Structure
  - Pathology.

- Treatment:
  - History of hypodontia
  - History of trauma
  - Unusual eruption pattern
  - Delayed appearance of teeth or unexplained missing teeth.
- Enforced extractions.
- Patient new to the practice.
- Referral for early orthodontics.

24.9 Clinical Justification for Taking Radiographs

According to the British Orthodontic Society (BOS) guidelines, clinicians have to have clinical justification for taking a radiograph.

According to the Ionising Radiation Medical Exposure Regulations 2000 (IR(ME)R 2000), clinicians have to keep exposure to a minimum.

24.9.1 Ionising Radiation Regulations

The Ionising Radiation Regulations (IRR 99) are concerned with the safety of those who work with ionising radiation. These regulations came into force on 1 January 2000 and replaced IRR 95.

IRR 99 contains the following safety requirements:

- The Health and Safety Executive must be informed of any radiographic equipment.
- The equipment must be regularly maintained and checked.
- There must be a radiation protection supervisor and a radiation advisor.
- There must be a designed controlled area.
- All operators must obey the local rules.
- A quality assurance programme must be in place (audit).

24.9.2 Ionising Radiation Medical Exposure Regulations

The IR(ME)R 2000 regulations came into force on 13 May 2000. This legislation sets out the responsibilities for duty holders (the employer, referrer, practitioner, and operator). It is also aimed at all patients to ensure their safety and protection against the hazards associated with ionising radiation.

The responsibilities that the duty holders have to ensure are:

- That all unintended, excessive, or incorrect medical exposures are minimised.
  - It is important to ensure that all medical exposures are minimised and that radiographs are not taken unnecessarily.
- That the benefit and the justification for the exposure outweigh the risk of the exposure.
  - Every radiograph taken must have a clinical justification for why it is needed and its benefit must outweigh the risks that it can have for the patient (e.g. exposure). No radiograph should be taken of a patient without a good enough clinical justification as to why that patient should be exposed to radiation.
- That all exposure doses are kept 'as low as reasonably practicable' during optimisation.
  - Everyone must have the correct exposure dose used on them and no excessive dose should be used at all when exposing the patient.

24.10   General Principles of Radiation

- Justification
  - Any exposure must have a benefit for the patient and outweigh the risks that the exposure can have for them.
  - No radiograph can be taken at any time without clinical justification.
- Optimisation
  - The exposure must be as low as possible.
  - The appropriate dose for the patient should be used.
  - No patient should be exposed to an excessive dose at any time.
- Limitation
  - The exposure must not exceed the limits recommended by the International Commission on Radiological Protection (ICRP).
- Radiation dosage:
  - Lateral cephalogram – 0.01 mSv.
  - DPT – 0.015–0.026 mSv.
  - Occlusal/periapical – 0.008 mSv.

25

Cephalometrics

A cephalometric or ceph radiograph is taken by use of the cephalostat. A ceph is a true lateral view of the skull, and is a two-dimensional image of a three-dimensional object, presenting an image of the skull and facial bones.

25.1 The Cephalostat

The cephalostat is an X-ray machine that takes cephalometric radiographs. It consists of ear posts that fit into the patient's external auditory meatus and a post, which helps stabilise the patient's head. When taking this X-ray the patient will be standing with their head positioned vertically and the Frankfort plane lying horizontally. The X-ray beam is directed to the ear posts and the distance from the tube to the patient is between 5 and 6 ft. (1.5–1.8 m) and from the patient to the film is around 1 ft. (30 cm).

25.2 Why Do We Take Cephalometrics?

Every cephalometric radiograph that is taken must always have a clinical justification. However, after clinical justification there are many reasons we would want to take a ceph:

- For cephalometric analysis:
  - This can either be evaluated by hand tracing or a digitiser.
- To work out:
  - Skeletal discrepancies in the anterio-posterior (AP) and vertical planes.
  - The angulation of the incisors.
- As an aid to diagnosis and treatment planning:
  - Cephs are not always part of a routine X-ray for patients going into treatment. However, they can constitute part of a pre-treatment record and are considered in patients who have a skeletal discrepancy and when anterio-posterior movement is planned for the upper and lower incisors.
- To monitor growth:
  - Cephs can be used to help monitor growth in patients, which is done by comparing and analysing two radiographs a year apart.

Textbook for Orthodontic Therapists, First Edition. Ceri Davies.
© 2020 John Wiley & Sons Ltd. Published 2020 by John Wiley & Sons Ltd.

- To monitor the progress of treatment:
  - Sometimes cephs can be used as part of monitoring the progress of treatment. However, this is very rarely done due to the clinical justification not being strong enough to outweigh the risks of exposure for the patient.
- To plan orthognathic surgery:
  - A ceph is considered in patients whose treatment involves orthognathic surgery (see Chapter 37). This type of X-ray can be used to help treatment planning for the surgery. It gives a representative image of the patient's skeletal features and assesses the true position of the maxilla and mandible.
- To assess the aetiology of malocclusion:
  - Cephs can also show the cause of the type of malocclusion the patient presents with. For example, a bimaxillary proclination could be considered as a class I incisor, but after analysing the ceph and evaluating the angulation of the incisors once they are at the correct angulation, the patient is in fact seen to be presenting with a skeletal class III discrepancy.
- To localise unerupted displaced teeth and any other pathology the patient could be presenting with.
- To measure growth changes in patients for study and research use.

25.3 When Do We Take a Cephalometric Radiograph?

Cephalometric radiographs can be considered after clinical examination has been done, but only when clinically justified. They are mainly used on patients with a skeletal discrepancy who require a two arch-fixed appliance or functional appliance.

25.4 Evaluating a Cephalometric Radiograph

Cephalometric radiographs always need to be evaluated, but first it is important to examine the radiograph for any abnormalities or pathology. Cephs are usually traced and there are two methods of doing this, hand tracing or by use of a digitiser.

25.4.1 Hand Tracing

Hand tracing is a task that is important, as it ensures use of the correct conditions and equipment. The following considerations should be employed:

- Hand tracing should be carried out by the use of a light viewing box in a darkened room, making it easier to see when plotting the points onto the ceph.
- Landmark identification is used on an acetate sheet which is laid over the film and should be secured by the use of masking tape to ensure it is in the same position as the patient was when the radiograph was taken (e.g. Frankfort plane horizontal).
- A sharp pencil must be used at all times when locating the landmark points.
- Stencils can be used to obtain a neat outline of the incisor and molar teeth.
- Landmark identification which is bilateral should be approached with care and an average of the two sides should be taken.
- Tracing errors should be of the order of:
  - +0.5 mm for linear measurements.
  - +0.5° for angular measurements.

25.4.2 Digitising

Cephalometric radiographs can also be traced by use of a digitiser when digital radiographs are taken. This is known to be as accurate as tracing by hand. Specialised software is needed for digital tracing and is achieved by the points being entered directly by the click of a mouse. Once this is done, it can be saved directly onto the patient's file.

25.4.3 Cephalometric Tracing Technique

Cephalometric tracing involves a special technique regardless of whether it is done by hand or on a digitiser. Failure to place the points in the correct position can result in the overall values being incorrect.

Tracing to construct a ceph analysis involves four different methods: drawing the soft tissue outline, placing the cephalometric points (landmark identification), constructing the planes and lines, and measuring the angles. Here we go into detail on how we construct a cephalometric analysis.

25.4.3.1 Draw a Soft Tissue Outline

Before beginning to trace a ceph, the following outlines should be drawn out by use of a sharp pencil:

- Forehead down towards the chin
- Sella turcica
- Forehead and nasal bone
- Orbitale
- Maxilla
- Mandible
- Upper and lower incisors.

25.4.3.2 Cephalometric Points

Once the soft tissue outline has been drawn, the following points are located on the ceph (Figure 25.1):

- Sella (S): the midpoint of the sella turcica.
- Porion (Por): the uppermost part of the external auditory meatus.
- Orbitale (Orb): the most anterior and inferior part of the margin of the orbit.
- Nasion (N): the most anterior point on the fronto-nasal suture.
- Anterior nasal spine (ANS): the tip of the ANS of the maxilla.
- Posterior nasal spine (PNS): the tip of the PNS of the maxilla.
- Gonion (Go): the most posterior and inferior point of the angle of the mandible.
  - The gonion can be guesstimated or determined more accurately by bisecting the angle formed by the tangents from the posterior border of the ramus and the inferior border of the mandible.
  - To construct the gonion:
    - o Draw tangents to the posterior and inferior borders.
    - o Bisect the angle formed by the tangents and mark where it crosses the angle of the mandible.
    - o Repeat for the other outline (if one is visible).
    - o The gonion is located midway between the two points.
- Menton (Me): the most inferior point on the mandibular symphysis.
- Pogonion (Pog): the most anterior point on the mandibular symphysis.
- Gnathian (Gna): the most anterior and inferior point on the mandibular symphysis.

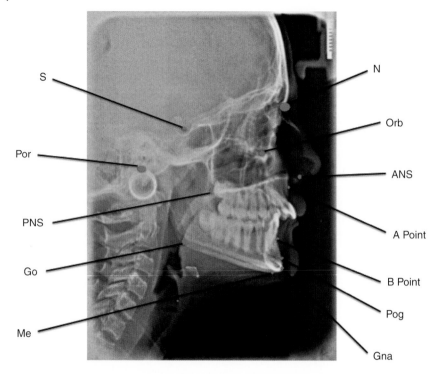

Figure 25.1 Where the landmark points are identified. For abbreviations see text.

- A Point: the deepest concavity on the anterior surface of the maxilla.
- B Point: the deepest concavity on the anterior surface of the mandible.

When the points have been plotted, the upper and lower incisor tip and apex are then located (Figure 25.2).

25.4.3.3 Cephalometric Planes and Lines
Once all the points are plotted the following lines are then drawn (Figure 25.3):

- SN line (Sella–Nasion), representing the cranial base.
- SNA line (Sella–Nasion–A Point).
- SNB line (Sella–Nasion–B Point).
- Frankfort plane (Orbitale–Porion).
- Maxillary plane (ANS–PNS).
- Mandibular plane (Gonion–Menton).
- Long axis of upper incisor.
- Long axis of lower incisor.
- Occlusal plane, drawn between the cusp tips of the permanent molars and premolars.
- A Pog (A Point–Pogonion).
- Perpendicular line (Nasion–Menton).

25.4.3.4 Measuring Angles
Once the points and lines have been drawn, the following angles are then measured by using a protractor:

- SNA: the angle where the SN line and A Point line meet.
- SNB: the angle where the SN line and B Point line meet.

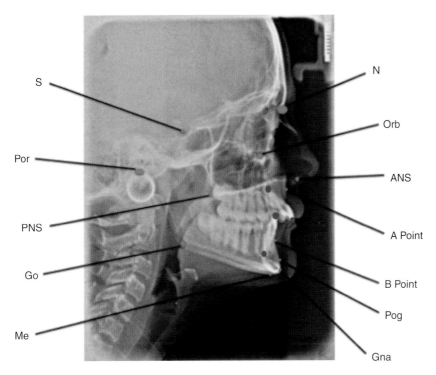

S

Por

PNS

Go

Me

N

Orb

ANS

A Point

B Point

Pog

Gna

Figure 25.2 Where the incisor apex and crown tip points are placed (in blue). For abbreviations see text.

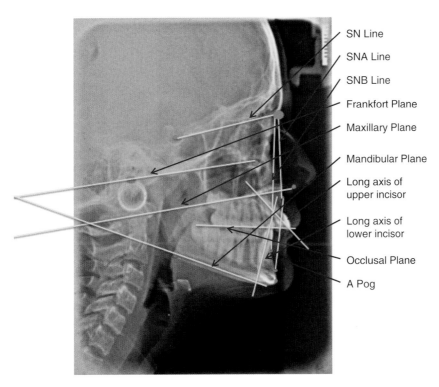

SN Line

SNA Line

SNB Line

Frankfort Plane

Maxillary Plane

Mandibular Plane

Long axis of
upper incisor

Long axis of
lower incisor

Occlusal Plane

A Pog

Figure 25.3 Cephalometric radiograph showing the cephalometric planes and lines. For abbreviations see text.

- ANB (SNA–SNB): the angle calculated by subtracting the angles of SNA and SNB.
- FMPA: the angle where the Frankfort and mandibular planes meet.
- MMPA: the angle where the maxillary and mandibular planes meet.
- Uinc to MxPl: the angle where the upper incisor line and maxillary plane meet.
- Linc to MnPl: the angle where the lower incisor line and mandibular plane meet.
- Interincisal (II): the angle where the lower incisor and upper incisor lines meet.
- Linc to Apog: a measurement in mm, calculated by the distance of where the lower incisor rests in relation to the Apog line.
- Facial proportion: the facial proportion percentage looks at both the upper and lower anterior facial heights and uses the maxillary plane angle. To work out the percentage the following calculation is used. Two perpendicular lines are drawn from the maxillary plane angle, one to the landmark point the menton (Me) and one to the nasion (N). The length of these lines is then measured in mm. The following calculation is used:

$$(MxPl - Me + MxPl - N) \div MxPl - Me \times 100$$

For example:
- Maxillary plane to mention (MxPl–Me) = 70 mm
- Maxillary plane to nasion (MxPl–N) = 57.5 mm
- MxPl–Me + MxPl–N = 70 + 57.5 = 127.5 mm
- 127.5 ÷ 70 × 100 = 54%

25.5 Eastman Analysis

Eastman analysis is a set of average values that help to construct a cephalometric analysis for Caucasians. The average values are shown in Table 25.1.

These values are used as a guideline that helps clinicians determine what angles a Caucasian would have if presenting with a skeletal class I discrepancy, an average vertical skeletal pattern, and the correct angulation of incisors. This helps clinicians to identify patients who have a skeletal class II or III pattern based on their angles against the normal average values that Eastman presents. For example, a patient with really proclined upper incisors is going to have an increased angle of more than 109°.

Table 25.1 Cephalometric average values for Caucasians (Eastman standard). For abbreviations see text.

SNA	81° +/− 3°
SNB	78° +/− 3°
ANB	3° +/− 2°
FMPA	28° +/− 4°
MMPA	27° +/− 4°
Uinc to MxPl	109° +/− 6°
Linc to MnPl	93° +/− 6°
II	135° +/− 10°
Linc to Apog	1 mm +/− 2 mm
Facial proportion	55% +/− 2%

25.6   ANB Angle

The ANB angle looks at the position of the maxilla and mandible, which helps to work out the patient's skeletal discrepancy in the AP plane. This is worked out by comparing the relationship of the maxilla and mandible with the cranial base by means of angles SNA and SNB.

The angle is then calculated by taking the difference of these two measurements away from each other. Doing this will calculate the ANB angle:

$$SNA - SNB = ANB$$

There are three categories of skeletal discrepancy when assessing the ANB angle:

- *Class I*: between 2° and 4°
- *Class II*: more than 4°
- *Class III*: less than 2°.

ANB correction is a technique that can be used to help work out the ANB angle. This is only considered when the nasion point is too far forward or back, which means the ANB angle will be incorrect. ANB correction helps to obtain a more accurate ANB angle.

- For every degree that SNA is below 81° (the average), add half a degree (0.5°) to ANB.
- For every degree that SNA is above 81° (the average), subtract half a degree (0.5°) from ANB.

For example, a tracing of a cephalometric radiograph results in an SNA angle of 75° and an ANB angle of 3°. However, from looking at the ceph the patient is clearly presenting with a skeletal class II discrepancy. ANB correction is needed:

- On the ceph, SNA = 75° and ANB = 3°
- 81° − 75° = 6°
- Add 3° to ANB angle 3° = 6° – class II skeletal.

For an overall understanding of how ANB correction works:

- Find the difference between the SNA angle and the Eastman analysis average 81° (81 – SNA).
- Halve the difference found between SNA and 81°.
- ANB +/− half the difference = ANB correction.
- If SNA below 81°, add the ANB correction.
- If SNA above 81°, subtract the ANB correction.

25.7   Wits Analysis and Ballard Conversion

There are two other approaches that can be used when working out the skeletal discrepancy in the AP plane: Wits analysis and Ballard conversion. Both avoid the use of the cranial base like the ANB angle does.

25.7.1   Wits Analysis

This method works out the skeletal discrepancy in the AP plane by comparing the relationship of the maxilla and mandible with use of the occlusal plane (Figure 25.4).

There are two steps in conducting this analysis:

1) The occlusal plane is drawn between the cusp tips of the molars and premolars (or deciduous molars).

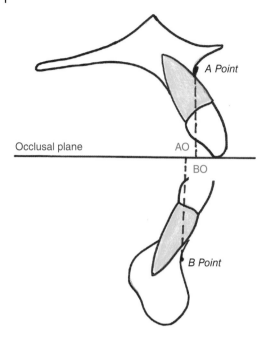

Figure 25.4 Wits analysis.

2) By use of the occlusal plane, two perpendicular lines are then dropped from A Point and B Point, which create two new points called AO and BO. The skeletal discrepancy is then determined by the position of AO and BO to one another.

The main disadvantage of using this approach is that the occlusal plane is not always easy to locate.

25.7.2 Ballard Conversion

This method works out the skeletal discrepancy in the AP plane by using the incisors to help work out the position of the maxilla and mandible by tipping the incisors into the average values of the Eastman analysis. This eliminates any dento-alveolar compensation and any residual overjet that remains will show the relationship of the maxilla and mandible.

The average values from the Eastman analysis are:

- Upper incisors 109° +/− 6°
- Lower incisors 93° +/− 6°.

To use the Ballard conversion, on a separate sheet of tracing paper trace the maxilla, mandibular symphysis, incisors, maxillary plane, and mandibular plane. Plot rotation points on the root one-third of the way from the root apex. By use of these rotation points, the upper incisors are rotated to 109° and the lower incisors to 93° from the maxilla and mandible. These are the average values from the Eastman analysis. Rotating them to the correct value will indicate any residual overjet, which will reflect the patient's true skeletal discrepancy (Figure 25.5).

25.8   Vertical Skeletal Pattern

The vertical skeletal pattern is worked out by use of the maxillary-mandibular plane angle (MMPA) and the Frankfort-mandibular plane angle (FMPA). This looks at how increased or decreased the lower anterior facial height (LAFH) is. However, most clinicians prefer to use the MMPA, as this is known to be easier to locate accurately.

- *MMPA*: this angle is located where the maxillary plane and mandibular plane meet. The average value from the Eastman analysis of Caucasians is 27° +/− 4°.
- *FMPA*: this angle is located where the Frankfort plane and mandibular plane meet. The average value from the Eastman analysis of Caucasians is 28° +/− 4°.

Patients with an *average* vertical skeletal pattern present with:

- Average values of FMPA (28°) and MMPA (27°).
- Seen in patients with a class I skeletal discrepancy.

Patients with an *increased* vertical skeletal pattern present with:

- Values higher than the average FMPA (+28°) and MMPA (+27°).
- Seen in patients with a class III skeletal discrepancy, increased LAFH, anterior openbite, and backward growth rotation.

Patients with a *decreased* vertical skeletal pattern present with:

- Values lower than the average FMPA (−28°) and MMPA (−27°).
- Seen in patients with a class II skeletal discrepancy, decreased LAFH, deepbite, and forward growth rotation.

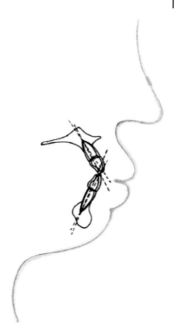

Figure 25.5   Ballard conversion. The incisors are traced and superimposed on their correct angles. This allows for the true skeletal pattern to be identified. Doing so allows the clinician to see the outcome of treatment as to where the incisors are going to be.

25.9   Angulation of the Incisors

The angles Uinc–MxPl and Linc–MnPl are used to help work out the angulation of the upper and lower incisors, with the use of the maxillary plane for the upper incisor and the mandibular plane for the lower incisor.

According to the Eastman analysis of Caucasians, the average values for these angles are:

- Uinc–MxPl = 109° +/− 6°
- Linc–MnPl = 93° +/− 6°.

If a patient presents with proclined upper incisors, the angle will probably be more than 109°; and vice versa, if the upper incisors are retroclined, the angle will be less than 109°.

If a patient presents with retroclined lower incisors, the angle will probably be less than 93°; and vice versa, if the lower incisors are proclined, the angle will be more than 93°.

25.10 Prognosis Tracing

Prognosis tracing is another method that can be used when incisor movement is planned by changing the angulation to correct an increased or reversed overjet. This is known as dento-alveolar compensation, as changing the incisors by proclining or retroclining them will show the patient's true skeletal pattern.

For a patient whose treatment is compromised, a prognosis tracing should be considered (Figure 25.6). It involves tracing the upper and lower incisors and changing their angulation values by tipping them or moving them bodily to work out the best course of treatment for the patient.

25.11 A-Pogonion Line (Apog)

Raleigh Williams, an orthodontist in the USA, created the Apog value, which is also known as the diagnostic line. This is the line that connects the A Point to the pogonion. From treating patients himself, Raleigh claimed that those who presented with pleasing facial appearances all had one thing in common, which was that the tip of their lower incisors lay on or just in front of the Apog line. For a good treatment goal, patients whose lower incisors finish in this position can ensure a good facial profile, although this is not an indication of good stability.

25.12 Cephalometric Errors

Errors can appear when constructing a ceph, and it is important to ensure that it is done correctly to prevent this. The most common errors that can occur are divided into three categories:

- *Projection errors*: a ceph is an enlarged two-dimensional representation of a three-dimensional object (the patient). Because of this angular measurements are preferred, as they are more accurate than linear measurements.

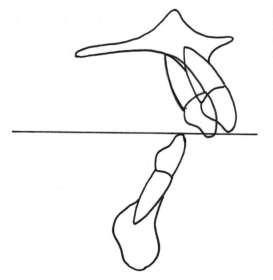

Figure 25.6 Prognosis tracing. This shows that bodily movement is not advisable to reduce an overjet, in this case due to the upper anterior segment being reduced out of the bone.

- *Landmark identification*: ensuring that landmark identification is accurate can be difficult if the radiograph is of poor quality. To prevent any errors in plotting the points, it is important to ensure that every clinician is using a sharp pencil. Blunt pencils can make the points bigger than they should be, which can result in the angular and linear measurements being incorrect.
- *Measurement errors*: incorrect plotting of landmark identifications can result in the angular measurements being incorrect and in some cases even multiplied.

26

Removable Appliances

A removable appliance is an orthodontic appliance that can be removed by the patient from the mouth for the maintenance of oral hygiene. Removables can either be an active appliance to aid tooth movement, or passive when prescribed as a retainer or as an appliance to maintain space within the arch.

26.1 Indications

Removables have many reasons for use and can be modified in so many ways. Indications for their use include:

- On upper and lower arches
- To produce tilting movements
- Overbite reduction
- Arch expansion
- Distal movement
- Space maintenance
- Stop digit sucking habit
- As an adjunct to fixed appliances
- For prefunctional phase of arch expansion and overbite reduction
- Eruption guidance
- As retainers.

26.2 Components

Removable appliances are made up of many components and the acronym ARAB helps remember all the different types:

A – Active components
R – Retentive components
A – Anchorage
B – Baseplate

Textbook for Orthodontic Therapists, First Edition. Ceri Davies.
© 2020 John Wiley & Sons Ltd. Published 2020 by John Wiley & Sons Ltd.

26.3 Active Components

These components are responsible for producing the desired tooth movement. This type of appliance can only produce tipping movement, when the tooth is tipped into its desired position around the tooth's centre of resistance. Active components are 0.5 mm thick and are constructed in hard polished stainless steel. To protect the components when in use, they are housed and embedded in the acrylic baseplate, which increases their support, preventing the chance of them deforming. There are many types of active components and they can come in the form of springs, screws, bows, and elastics.

26.3.1 Springs

Palatal finger spring (Figure 26.1):

- Is fabricated in 0.5 mm diameter stainless steel.
- Allows distal movement of canines, premolars, and molars.
- If overactivated can result in excessive tipping of the teeth.

Buccal canine retractor (Figure 26.2):

- Is fabricated in 0.5 mm diameter stainless steel.
- Allows palatal and distal movement of mesially and labially angulated canines.

Z spring or double cantilever spring (Figure 26.3):

- Allows labial movement.
- Is fabricated in 0.5 mm diameter stainless steel.
- Allows proclination of one or two incisors.
- Is activated by pulling away from baseplate at 45°.

T spring (Figure 26.4):

- Allows labial movement.
- Is fabricated in 0.5 mm stainless steel.

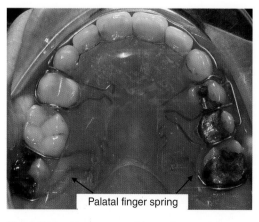

Figure 26.1 Upper removable appliance with palatal finger springs.

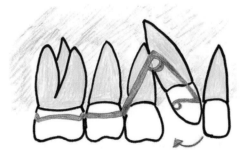

Figure 26.2 Buccal canine retractor.

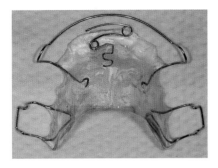

Figure 26.3 Upper removable appliance with Z spring.

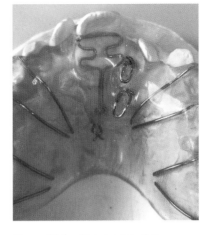

Figure 26.4 Upper removable appliance with T spring.

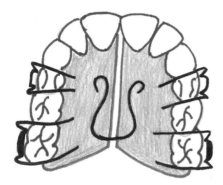

Figure 26.5 Coffin spring.

- Allows proclination of an incisor, canine, premolar, or molar.
- Is activated by pulling away from baseplate at 45°.

Coffin spring (Figure 26.5):

- Allows for expansion in the upper arch.
- Is fabricated in 1.25 mm diameter stainless steel.
- Corrects buccal crossbites.
- Is an alternative to midline expansion screw.

Recurved spring:

- Allows proclination of all four incisors.
- Allows labial movement.
- Is fabricated in 0.8 mm diameter stainless steel.

Crossover wires:

- Allow labial movement.
- Are fabricated in 0.7–0.8 mm diameter stainless steel.
- Allow proclination of all four incisors.

26.3.1.1 Equation for Springs

When placing force to teeth via springs, it is important to consider the equation involved. This equation works out the force the spring is applying dependent on the deflection radius and the length of the wire involved. The following equation is considered when springs are being activated and designed:

$$F = dr^4 / L^3$$

where F = force; d = distance of deflection; r = radius; L = length.

- Doubling the radius of the wire increases the force 16-fold and doubling the length of the wire decreases the force 8-fold.
- Increasing the length of the wire and/or reducing the thickness (diameter) of the wire results in lighter forces.
- Reducing the length of the wire and/or increasing the thickness (diameter) of the wire results in heavier forces.
- However, increasing the length of the wire and/or reducing the thickness (diameter) of the wire will make the spring more susceptible to distortion and breakage.

26.3.2 Screws

Screws are another active component that can be used to move blocks or groups of teeth only. There are three types of screws that can be used: anterior expansion screw, midline expansion screw, and a combination of the two known as a 3D expansion screw.

All screws are made from stainless steel, the same as springs, and they are compromised into two halves and joined together by use of a threaded central cylinder. Activation of the screws is by use of a key that is turned a quarter turn once a week, resulting in 0.25 mm of movement, creating 1 mm of movement a month.

Anterior expansion screw (Figure 26.6):

- Allows labial movement.
- Corrects anterior crossbites by proclination of multiple incisors.
- Is used to push a block of teeth at a time.
- Is adjusted by a key, with one quarter turn per week resulting 0.25 mm of movement.
- Consists of two halves joined together by a central cylinder.

Midline expansion screw (Figure 26.7):

- Allows expansion of the upper arch.
- Allows two blocks of teeth to be moved to correct posterior buccal crossbites.
- Adjusted by a key, with one quarter turn per week resulting in 0.25 mm of movement.
- Consists of two halves and a threaded central cylinder.

3D expansion screw (Figure 26.8):

- Combines both an anterior expansion screw and a midline expansion screw.
- Proclines the anterior segment and expands the posterior segment in the upper arch.
- Is adjusted by turning the key one day for the midline expansion screw and two to three days later for the anterior expansion screw.
- Both screws are activated on different days of the week to prevent confusion for the patient.

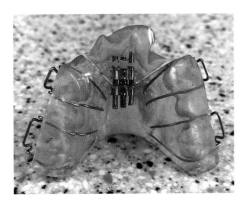

Figure 26.6 Upper removable appliance with anterior expansion screw.

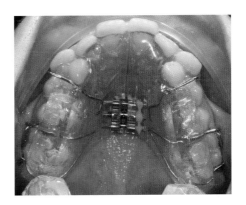

Figure 26.7 Upper removable appliance with midline expansion screw.

Figure 26.8 Upper removable appliance with 3D expansion screw.

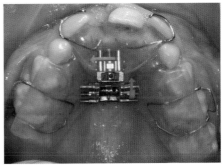

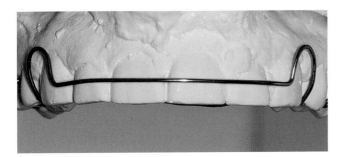

Figure 26.9 Active labial bow on study model.

26.3.3 Active Bows

When considering a bow for a removable appliance, the majority of people may consider a labial bow as just a retentive component; however, it can also be used as an active component. There are two types of active bows, both made out of stainless steel ranging from 0.5 to 0.7 mm. The orthodontist achieves activation of these bows using Adams spring-forming pliers.

Active labial bow (Figure 26.9):

- Is constructed in 0.7mm stainless steel.
- Is used to retract the upper incisors if there is an increased overjet.
- Creates tipping.

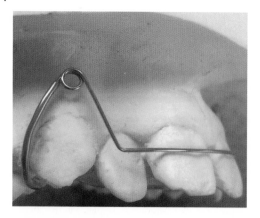

Figure 26.10   Right buccal view of Roberts retractor.

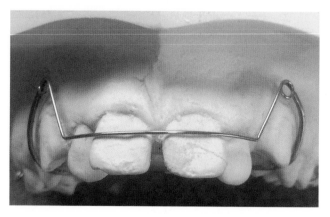

Figure 26.11   Centre view of Roberts retractor.

Roberts retractor (Figures 26.10 and 26.11):

- Allows palatal movement.
- Is fabricated in 0.5 mm diameter stainless steel inserted into stainless-steel tubing.
- Allows retraction of proclined and spaced maxillary incisors.
- Is activated using Adams spring-forming pliers by twisting circular inserts on the Roberts retractor.

26.3.4   Elastics

Intra-oral elastics are another type of active component that can be used and are mainly considered to move individual teeth. These elastics would be considered for intrusion, extrusion, and palatal movement. When referring to palatal movement, a palatally displaced canine can be brought into alignment via a button and elastic. All elastics come in different sizes and can range from 2, 3.5, to 4.5 oz. Options of latex or latex-free elastics can be considered, especially for patients who suffer from a latex allergy. Stretching elastic to three times its original size activates it to achieve application of the full force.

Advantages of elastics:

- Good aesthetics.
- They have the ability to apply intrusive and extrusive movements.

Disadvantages of elastics:

- The force level diminishes rapidly intra-orally.
- They often snap during use.

Examples of intrusion and extrusion with elastics:

- *Intrusion with elastics*: Intrusion of teeth can be achieved on a removable appliance. For example, if UR1 needs intruding, by bonding a button incisally and running elastic from the button to the labial bow, this creates a vertical component of force that will allow intrusion.
- *Extrusion with elastics*: extrusion of teeth can be achieved on a removable appliance. For example, if an impacted maxillary central incisor needs extruding, by bonding a button onto the tooth and having the labial bow modified with helices, an elastic can be attached from the button to the helices on the labial bow, which will create a vertical component of force to allow extrusion of this tooth.

26.3.5 Headgear

Headgear is an orthodontic appliance that is used extra-orally (outside the mouth). As well as being in use with fixed appliances, it can also be used with a removable appliance and can be used for extra-oral anchorage and extra-oral traction. Extra-oral anchorage only achieves distal movement of the molars, while extra-oral traction achieves distal movement of molars, intrusion, extrusion, maxillary restraint, correction of crossbites, and reduction in overjet. However, nowadays headgear is rarely used, especially with removables, as one of its disadvantages is that the headgear can distort and cause breakages to the Adams clasp.

Headgear has three different types of pull which all achieve different movements (Figure 26.12). High pull headgear:

- Achieves:
  - Distalisation of molars
  - Intrusion of molars
  - Maxillary restraint.
- Forces transmitted above occlusal plane.

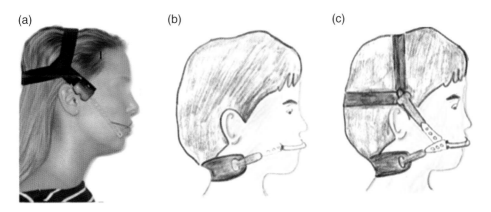

Figure 26.12 Three different pulls of headgear: (a) high pull; (b) cervical (low) pull; (c) straight (Interlandi or combi) pull.

- Used in patients with:
  - Class III malocclusion
  - Anterior overbite (AOB) with increased maxillary-mandibular plane angle (MMPA)
  - Backward growth rotation.

Cervical pull (low pull) headgear:

- Achieves
  - Distalisation of molars
  - Extrusion of molars.
- Forces transmitted below occlusal plane.
- Used in patients with:
  - Class II
  - Deepbite/increased overbite
  - Forward growth rotation.

Straight pull (Interlandi or combi-pull) headgear:

- Achieves distalisation of molars with extra-oral appliances.
- Contains both low and high pull.
- Forces transmitted level with occlusal plane.

Attaching the facebow to a removable appliance can be done in two ways. Adams clasps (see next section) can be made with a soldered bridge on them which allows the facebow to be locked into it, or J hooks can be used which allow the facebow to lock into the U loops.

26.4   Retentive Components

Retentive components make up an essential part of a removable appliance. As well as enabling the active components to work efficiently, they help with seating of the appliance in the mouth and aid in patient comfort. These components are made out of 0.7 mm stainless steel and are slightly thicker than the active components, due to the good strength they need to have from the numerous adjustments that are made throughout treatment.

Many different retentive components can be used on a removable appliance, such as the Adams clasp, Southend clasp, C clasp, ball-ended clasp, labial bow, and Plint clasp.

Adams clasp (Figures 26.13 and 26.14):

- Is also known as an arrowhead clasp.
- Is most commonly used on premolars and molars.
- Is engaged at the mesial and distal gingival undercuts.
- Buccal bars (bridge) are helpful for removal and placement for the patient.

Southend clasp (Figure 26.15):

- Is used for anterior retention.
- Is used on upper central incisors or just a central and lateral incisor, depending on the design for retention.
- The clasp is bent back towards the labial undercut just below the gingival margin for maximum hold.
- The disadvantage of this clasp is its visibility.

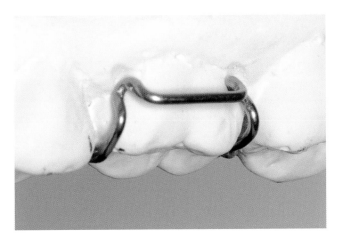

Figure 26.13   Adams clasp.

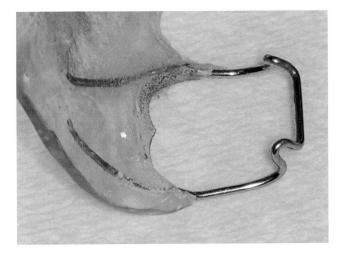

Figure 26.14   Adams clasp.

C clasp (Figure 26.16):

- Is used to engage the interproximal gingival undercut of canines and molars.
- The advantage of the clasp is the possibility of avoiding occlusal interference on one side.

Ball-ended clasp (Figure 26.17):

- Is commonly used between the lower incisors for anterior retention or the upper premolars, especially when a removable appliance is used in conjunction with a fixed appliance.
- Interproximal spacing can occur due to the clasps being engaged by the interproximal undercuts.
- Is bent towards the undercuts for a good hold.
- Crosses the occlusal/incisal surface between two adjacent teeth and engages the mesiobuccal and distobuccal undercuts.

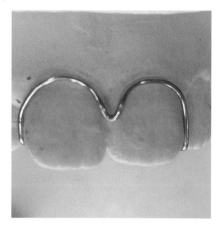

Figure 26.15 Southend clasp.

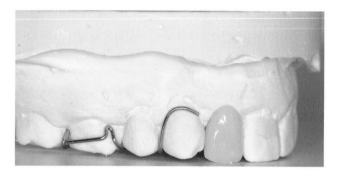

Figure 26.16 Upper removable appliance with C clasp over UR3 and pontic in place for missing UR2.

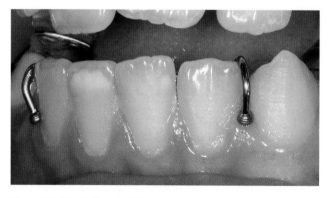

Figure 26.17 Ball-ended clasps over lower anterior teeth used for anterior retention.

Labial bow (Figure 26.18):

- Can be used as an active or retentive component.
- Lies on the labial surface of teeth and can be good anterior retention for holding the incisor position.
- When used as an active component, can help reduce an overjet by squeezing the U loops using Adams pliers.

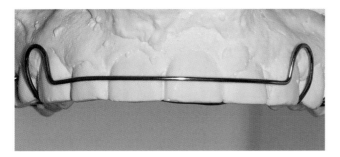

Figure 26.18 Retentive labial bow on study model.

- Can be used on a Hawley retainer for retention purposes to maintain the position of teeth and prevent relapse.
- For retention purposes, modification of the labial bow can be achieved by bending the wire to contour the teeth or by adding acrylic, shaped around the teeth, for maximum hold, which is known as an acrylated labial bow.
- The main disadvantage of a labial bow is its high visibility.

Plint clasp:

- Is used when maxillary molar bands are in place.
- Engages the undercuts and into the tube of the molar band.
- Consideration for their use is when a removable appliance is used in conjunction with fixed appliances and headgear.

26.5 Anchorage

During orthodontic treatment with any type of appliance, anchorage is very important, as it is the resistance to unwanted tooth movement. Anchorage can maintain the extraction space by preventing the upper molars from moving mesially and hold the expansion of the arch which has been created. On a removable appliance anchorage comes from the acrylic baseplate, which provides a good source of anchorage in all three planes of space, antero-posterior, vertical, and transverse. The reason an acrylic baseplate maintains a good source of anchorage is because the forces from the appliance transmit across the baseplate, unwanted forces are dissipated over the palatal tissues, many teeth can be included in the anchor unit, and any active forces can be kept light.

To increase anchorage, headgear can also be used with a removable appliance, providing extra-oral anchorage to prevent molars from moving mesially and help with maxillary restraint. The accurate colletting on a removable appliance is also a good source of anchorage. This is found where the acrylic from the baseplate sits around the gingival margin (Figure 26.19). It helps the acrylic baseplate hold the arch width and maintain the tooth positions.

26.6 Baseplate

The baseplate on a removable appliance can be made from two types of acrylic material. Self-cure/cold cure acrylic, known as polymethacrylate, is the most popular material to use on a removable appliance. Heat cure acrylic can be used, but is more likely to be considered on a

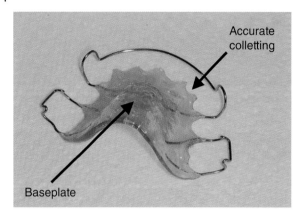

Figure 26.19 Upper removable appliance with labial bow and Adams clasps.

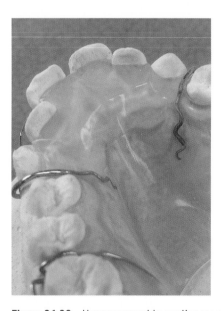

Figure 26.20 Upper removable appliance with flat anterior bite plane.

functional appliance, which is more robust, comes under more strain, and needs heightened strength from the bite blocks.

The baseplate can be active or passive and has many functions:

- It anchors teeth, preventing unwanted tooth movement.
- The forces applied by the appliance are transmitted across the palate.
- It houses all the active and retentive components, protecting them from any damage.

Bite planes can also be incorporated within the baseplate, such as a flat anterior bite plane (FABP), a posterior bite plane, also known as occlusal capping, and an inclined anterior bite plane.

Flat anterior bite plane (Figure 26.20):

- Is found on the anterior segment of the baseplate, by the palatal surface of the incisors.
- Is considered in deepbite cases as it is used for the reduction of overbites.

- Creates incisor intrusion in the lower and lower passive molar eruption.
- Can be manufactured at any time, either when the appliance is made or added throughout treatment at a later stage, depending on the type of case.
- The wedge effect principle is associated with the patient's bite by using the MMPA. For example, increasing the wedge effect will open up the patient's bite by allowing passive lower molar eruption, useful in deepbite cases; whereas in anterior openbite cases, by decreasing the wedge effect you intrude the posterior segment, which will help to close the bite down.
- The height of an FABP should be half the height of the upper central incisors, so that it disarticulates the posterior segment by 1–3 mm between the upper and lower molars. However, during manufacturing this should be taken with care, because if the bite plane is too high it may interfere with patient compliance.

Posterior bite plane (Figure 26.21):

- Is found on the occlusal surfaces of the posterior segment and works in the same way as glass ionomer cement (GIC) bite blocks during fixed appliance treatment.
- Occlusal capping is another name for the posterior bite plane.
- Helps open the patient's bite, reducing any occlusal interferences from other teeth that may interfere with the correction of anterior and posterior crossbites.
- Is only prescribed when elimination of any occlusal interferences is needed and reduction of the overbite is undesired (not wanted).
- Manufacturing of a posterior bite plane involves the baseplate carrying the acrylic over to the occlusal surfaces of the buccal posterior segment. This will prop the bite open, relieving any occlusal interferences.
- Care should be taken during manufacture to ensure the bite plane is not too thick, as this will help with patient tolerance.

Inclined anterior bite plane:

- Is found on the palatal surface in the upper anterior segment.
- Is used after functional appliance treatment, as it holds the lower jaw in the correct position and maintains the incisor relationship.

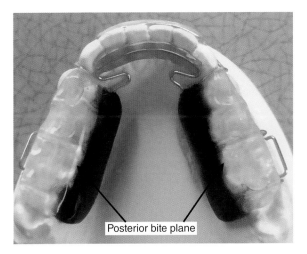

Figure 26.21 Lower removable appliance with posterior bite planes.

- Looks identical to an FABP; however, this type has small grooves within the acrylic of the bite plane behind the upper incisors where the patient bites, maintaining the correct lower jaw position.
- Also helps to correct a deepbite, as it still disarticulates the posterior segment, allowing for passive lower molar eruption.

26.7   Advantages and Disadvantages of Removable Appliances

Advantages:

- Can be removed for oral hygiene purposes.
- Anchorage is increased due to the palatal coverage from the baseplate.
- Easy to adjust for clinicians.
- Acrylic can be added to form bite planes at any time before and during treatment.
- Can be used for retentive purposes and as a space maintainer.
- Can be used to transmit forces for individual teeth or blocks of teeth.
- There is less risk of iatrogenic damage (root resorption).
- Can be used for interceptive treatment for early crossbites in mixed dentition.
- Inexpensive.

  Disadvantages:

- Can be left out, resulting in compliance issues with the patient.
- Can only achieve tipping movement of teeth, no bodily movement.
- Requires a good technician.
- Can affect speech.
- A lower appliance can result in a tolerance issue for patients.
- Inefficient at multiple tooth movements.

26.8   Stages of Removable Appliances

A patient will first come into the practice for a consultation with the prescribing orthodontist for a clinical assessment to discuss treatment options. Once the patient has been prescribed a removable appliance, they will go through the following stages, from records to post-removable treatment, which can involve orthodontic therapists.

- Chairside:
  - Records appointment.
  - Records taken: X-rays, photos and impressions.
  - Design of appliance on laboratory form, sent with impressions.
- Lab:
  - Construction: appliance is made from impressions sent to the lab.
- Fit and instructions:
  - Fit appliance.
  - Active components are activated by the orthodontist, but orthodontic therapists can fit them and adjust non-active components.

- Review – monitor and activate:
  - Monitor patient at every appointment – points to check:
    o If patient has been wearing the appliance.
    o Whether they can put it in.
    o Any indentation of soft tissues on palate.
    o Tooth wear on acrylic due to eating with the appliance in.
    o Lisp with speech.
    o Whether teeth are moving.

26.9 Instruments Used on a Removable Appliance

- Adams pliers: to adjust retentive components.
- Spring-forming pliers: to activate active components.
- Mauns wire cutters.
- Dividers: to measure space, for example expansion of the upper arch from midline expansion screw.
- Ruler.
- Straight handpiece and acrylic bur: to adjust acrylic.

26.10 Fitting of a Removable Appliance

Points to consider when fitting a removable appliance:

- Check prescription is correct.
- Show appliance to patient and explain how it works.
- Check for roughness on fitting surface.
- Try the appliance in (the orthodontist activates the active components).
- Show patient how to insert and remove, get patient to practise.
- Give patient instructions for use.

27

Functional Appliances

A functional appliance can be a fixed or a removable appliance that is used in class II malocclusions that achieves a forward posture of the mandible, causing stretching of the facial soft tissues to produce a combination of dental and skeletal changes. Of these changes,
70% are dento-alveolar and 30% are skeletal.

27.1 Timing of Treatment

Functional appliance treatment is not suitable for everyone and can only be used on specific patients. The ideal patient for functional treatment is an actively growing patient, because coinciding with their pubertal growth spurt gives maximum effect of movement. The ideal age for girls is between the ages of 10–12 years, as they stop growing at 16, and for boys is between the ages of 14 and 16 years, as they stop growing at 18. It is best for the patient to be in the late mixed dentition, as this will allow for a smooth transition from functional to fixed appliance treatment. Earlier treatment can be considered if there is a risk of trauma, such as the patient having a 10+ mm overjet or due to psychological reasons such as bullying or teasing at school.

27.2 Malocclusion Types

There are only certain malocclusion types that can be used with functional appliance treatment. The malocclusions considered are class II div I, class II div II, and class III cases; however, class III cases are rarely treated with functional appliances nowadays.

27.2.1 Class II Div I

To correct a class II div I case with a functional appliance:

- Appliance must be worn full time for an average of six to eight months.
- Appliance will posture the mandible forward to achieve a working bite.
- Posturing the mandible forward will reduce the increased overjet. The ideal overjet at the end of treatment is 0 mm.

Textbook for Orthodontic Therapists, First Edition. Ceri Davies.
© 2020 John Wiley & Sons Ltd. Published 2020 by John Wiley & Sons Ltd.

- Incisors to be class III or edge to edge at the end.
- Molars will be class III.
- Canines will be class III.
- Once these corrections have been achieved with a functional appliance, the patient will then follow on to fixed appliances to close the bite down and correct individual tooth movement.

27.2.2   Class II Div II

A class II div II is treated slightly differently and has three stages. A different treatment approach is considered before a patient goes into a functional appliance.

- Stage 1: the patient begins with one of these three treatment options:
  - Upper removable appliance (URA) with Z spring or anterior expansion screw to procline incisors to class II div I.
  - Upper sectional fixed U2-2 to procline incisors to class II div I.
  - Functional appliance incorporating an active component such as a Z spring. This helps by posturing the mandible forward to achieve a working bite, at the same time as the incisors are being proclined to class II div I.
- Stage 2: once the proclination of the upper anterior incisors is achieved, the patient is then treated the same as a class II div I case:
  - A functional appliance to posture the lower mandible forward to achieve a working bite by reducing the overjet and achieving class III incisors, canines, and molars.
- Stage 3: once a working bite is achieved, the patient will follow on to fixed appliance treatment to close the bite down and correct individual tooth movement.

27.2.3   Class III

Treating a class III case with a functional appliance is rarely done nowadays. There are only two types of functional appliances that can be used to help in the correction of a class III case.

- Reverse Clark's twin block:
  - Used to help retract the mandible. The lower bite block comes behind the upper bite block.
- Frankel regulator 3 (FR3):
  - Used to retract the mandible and eliminate cheek pressure by the acrylic buccal shields, which allow for upper arch expansion, correcting any buccal crossbites.

27.3   The End Point

The end point is very important when it comes to functional appliance treatment. Overcorrecting the patient is always considered, as this allows for some relapse to happen during the transition stage from functional to fixed appliance treatment.

The features seen after functional treatment are:

- Reduced overjet 0 mm (edge to edge)
- Class III molars
- Class III incisors
- Class III canines.

27.4 Ten Key Points of Functional Appliances

1) Used in actively growing patients.
2) Posture the mandible forward.
3) Used in late mixed dentition.
4) Can be used for psychological reasons.
5) Worth a try in any class II case.
6) Usually followed by fixed appliances.
7) Can be used alone if arches are well aligned – rare.
8) Produce mainly dento-alveolar changes.
9) Response varies between patients.
10) Difficult to wear, need a lot of encouragement.

27.5 Indications for Treatment

Patients who present with the following indications should be considered for functional appliance treatment:

- Mild to moderate skeletal II case.
- Increased overjet.
- Reduced lower anterior facial height (LAFH) or average LAFH.
- Proclined maxillary incisors.
- Retroclined mandibular incisors.
- Actively growing patient.
- Class II molars/canines.

27.6 Mode of Action

The mode of action describes how the appliance works. These are the key points of what is achieved on patients who have a functional appliance:

- Dento-alveolar changes (70% of changes):
  - Retroclined maxillary incisors.
  - Proclined mandibular incisors.
  - Distal movement of upper dentition.
  - Mesial movement of lower dentition.
- Increase in mandibular length – skeletal changes (30% of changes):
  - Downward and forward translation of the condyle.
  - Encouraging compensatory backward growth of the condyle.
- Increased LAFH:
  - Passive molar eruption.
  - Backward mandibular growth.
- Forward remodelling of the glenoid fossa.
- Maxillary restraint:
  - Due to class II traction forces.
  - Incorporation with headgear.

27.7 Advantages and Disadvantages of Functionals

Advantages:

- Can be removed for oral hygiene purposes.
- Anchorage is increased due to the palatal coverage from the baseplate.
- Easy to adjust for clinicians.
- Less risk of iatrogenic damage.

  Disadvantages:

- Appliance can be left out, resulting in compliance issues with the patient.
- Can only achieve tipping movement of teeth, no bodily movement.
- Requires a good technician.
- Appliance can affect speech.
- Lower appliance can result in a tolerance issue for patients.
- Appliance can cause gingival trauma.
- Appliance can cause jaw ache.
- Appliance can cause muscle ache.

27.8 Types of Functional Appliances

There are six different types of functional appliances, which all achieve the same type of movement. They are categorised into different groups:

- *Tissue borne*: meaning the appliance is fitted and retained in place by the soft tissues.
- *Tooth borne*: meaning the appliance is fitted and retained in place by the teeth.
- *Removable*: meaning the functional appliance is removable.
- *Fixed*: meaning the functional appliance is fixed to the teeth.

27.8.1 Clark's Twin Block

The Clark's twin block appliance (Figures 27.1 and 27.2) was designed by Dr William Clark and is the most popular appliance used today because it is well tolerated by patients. It is a removable tooth-borne appliance, meaning it can be removed from the mouth by the patient and is retained in place by the teeth. It is also known as a two-piece functional appliance due to having two parts (an upper and a lower). The twin block can be modified to help correct the arch in the antero-posterior, vertical, and transverse planes.

27.8.1.1 How Does It Work?

- The upper and lower parts fit together by using posterior bite blocks which are 7–8 mm high. The lower bite block comes in front of the upper bite block. The bite blocks interlock with each other and help posture the mandible forward. The bite blocks interdigitate at 70°.
- The appliance must be worn full time, including when eating; it must be removed for contact sports and cleaning teeth, but should go straight back in.

Figure 27.1 Clark's twin block in full interdigitation.

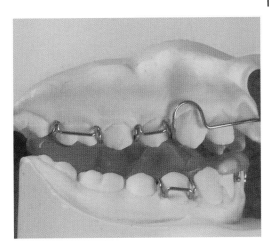

Figure 27.2 Clark's twin block not in full interdigitation.

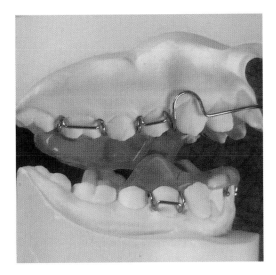

- The appliance can allow upper arch expansion with a midline expansion screw or be modified to allow proclination of the upper incisors in class II div II cases with an anterior expansion screw or Z spring, which can be housed within the acrylic baseplate.
- Some clinicians like to achieve more of a skeletal change, therefore modifying the lower twin block by placing acrylic coverage over the lower incisors will help do this (Figure 27.3).

27.8.1.2 Effects of Clark's Twin Blocks

Many effects on the dentition come with wearing twin blocks:

- Posterior lateral openbites, seen especially in patients with deepbites.
- The posterior teeth may be unerupted or erupted due to the occlusal coverage of the bite blocks. The acrylic bite blocks stop the posterior teeth from erupting. Some clinicians will trim the acrylic away from occlusal surfaces of the block to allow the lower molars to erupt.
- Any remaining lateral openbites are closed down in the fixed appliance stage.

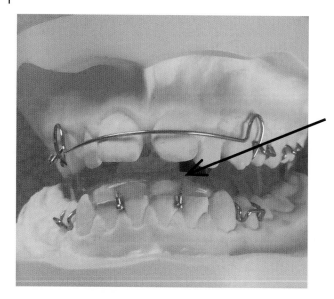

Figure 27.3 Clark's twin block with acrylic coverage on lower incisors. Acrylic coverage on lower incisors (arrow) prevents proclination of lower incisors, allowing for more of a skeletal change than a dento-alveolar change.

27.8.1.3 Advantages

- Patient can move mandible, making it easier to speak and eat with the appliance in.
  For aesthetics the appliance makes:
  - Immediate improvement in appearance.
  - No labial bow means appliance cannot be seen.
- Appliance being worn full time means it works fast and efficiently.
- Appliance can be integrated with fixed appliances – at the same time or post-functional appliance.
- Is a two-piece functional appliance with separate upper and lower parts.
- Is well tolerated by patients.
- Can be modified by screws and springs to correct the upper arch in the antero-posterior and transverse planes.
- If worn really well can result in rapid treatment changes.
- Is easy to adjust and reactivate.

27.8.1.4 Disadvantages

- Patients need to have a lot of encouragement to wear the appliance.
- The desired end result will not be achieved if it is not worn.
- At first the appliance is difficult to wear.
- If worn during eating this results in more cleaning of the appliance after meals.
- Each patient's response can vary, some get on well with the appliance but some do not.
- Lower anterior facial height (LAFH) is increased, so it is to be used with caution if patients already present with an increased LAFH/FMPA (Frankfort-mandibular plane angle).
- Occlusal rests are found on 7s.
- Results in lateral openbites.

27.8.2 Herbst Appliance

The Herbst appliance (Figure 27.4) was developed in 1905 by a German orthodontist called Dr Emil Herbst. It is a fixed functional appliance and is tooth borne, meaning it attaches to the teeth. The best advantage of this appliance is that it is non-compliance dependent: because it is fixed to the teeth, it is constantly working and patients do not have to remember to insert and remove it. Even though the twin block appliance is well tolerated by patients, the Herbst is known to be even better tolerated: it is less bulky than the twin block, which makes it easier to speak and eat with it in place.

27.8.2.1 How Does It Work?

- There are two sections: one section attaches to the upper buccal segment teeth and the other to the lower buccal segment teeth.
- The two sections are then joined by a rigid arm that is activated and this postures the mandible forwards.
- Reducing overjets with this appliance is just as successful as with twin blocks.

27.8.2.2 Advantages

- Works efficiently as it is fixed to the teeth and cannot be removed.
- Is well tolerated by patients.
- Is good for aesthetics due to the appliance being attached on the posterior segments, making it hardly seen.
- Easier to talk and eat with appliance in.

27.8.2.3 Disadvantages

- Increased breakages can occur.
- Higher cost.

Figure 27.4 Herbst appliance.

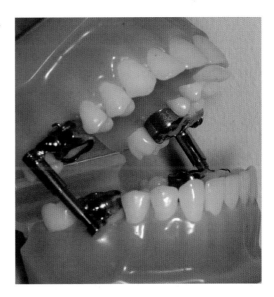

- Difficult to use.
- Difficult to repair.
- Expensive.

27.8.3 Medium Opening Activator

The medium opening activator (MOA; Figures 27.5 and 27.6) was developed in 1908 by Viggo Anderson and was the first widely used functional appliance. It can be removed by the patient and is retained in place by the teeth, making it a removable tooth-borne functional appliance. It differs from the twin block, as it is a one-piece functional appliance, which means the patient is unable to eat or speak with it in place. There is minimal acrylic on the appliance and not only does it improve patient comfort but, due to no molar capping, it allows for posterior molar eruption. This works well in a deepbite case, as this will help to open the bite.

27.8.3.1 How Does It Work?

- The upper and lower parts are joined together by two rigid acrylic posts.
- Between the rigid acrylic posts is an anterior breathing hole.

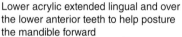

Lower acrylic extended lingual and over the lower anterior teeth to help posture the mandible forward

Figure 27.5 Medium opening activator appliance.

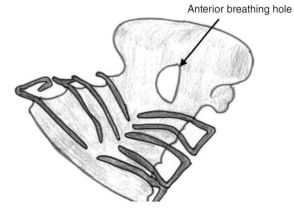

Lower teeth

No lower molar capping allowing posterior molar eruption

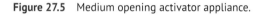

Anterior breathing hole

Figure 27.6 Occlusal (upside-down) view of a medium opening activator.

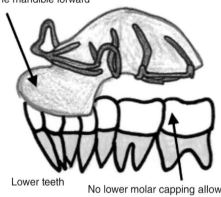

- On the lower part, the acrylic extends lingually to the lower labial segment; this area contains grooves within the acrylic where the lower teeth sit. This helps posture the mandible forward and holds it in the desired position.

27.8.3.2 Advantages

- Contains a breathing hole anteriorly.
- Contains minimal acrylic.
- No molar capping, allowing teeth to erupt freely – good for deepbite cases.
- Is less bulky.
- Can be modified with fixed appliances.

27.8.3.3 Disadvantages

- Is a one-piece functional appliance.
- Is difficult to tolerate.
- Patient cannot speak with appliance in.
- Patient cannot eat with appliance in, which prevents appliance working fast and efficiently.

27.8.4 Bionator Appliance

Wilhelm Balters developed the bionator appliance in 1964. It is a one-piece functional appliance that can be removed by the patient (Figure 27.7). The bionator is retained in the mouth by the teeth and soft tissues, making it both tooth and tissue borne. The two main advantages of this appliance are that it is easy to clean due to it being removable and it contains less acrylic, meaning it reduces lisping for the patient, especially in the palate. However, even though the appliance can be removed for cleaning, this also leads to a disadvantage as it prevents the appliance from working fast and efficiently, as it has to be removed if the patient wants to speak or eat. Originally the appliance was designed to modify tongue behaviour by use of the heavy wire loop incorporated in the palate. As well as modifying tongue behaviour. the heavy wire loop, also known as a coffin spring, can help expand the upper arch.

27.8.4.1 How Does It Work?

- The labial bow extends buccally and these extensions of the bow hold the cheeks out of the way, stopping any contact with the buccal segment teeth. This allows for some arch expansion.

Figure 27.7 Bionator appliance.

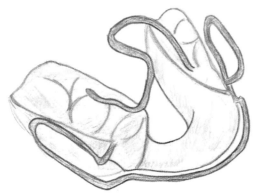

- Grooves are found in the lower acrylic where the lower incisor edges occlude; this helps to posture the mandible forward and hold it in the desired position.
- The posterior part of the appliance contain acrylic blocks that the teeth bite onto by the grooves in the acrylic.

27.8.4.2 Advantages

- Is removable, making it easier to clean.
- Reduces lisping due to less acrylic in the palate.

27.8.4.3 Disadvantages

- Is a one-piece functional appliance.
- Patient is unable to speak or eat with appliance in, which prevents appliance working fast and efficiently.
- Posterior acrylic blocks prevent molars erupting.

27.8.5 Frankel Appliance

Rolf Frankel developed the Frankel appliance in the 1950s, also known as the Frankel functional regulator. It is a one-piece functional removable appliance and can be removed by the patient (Figure 27.8). The Frankel is the only completely tissue-borne appliance, meaning it is only retained in the mouth by the soft tissues.

There are three types of functional regulator:

- FR1 to treat class II div I
- FR2 to treat class II div II
- FR3 to treat class III.

27.8.5.1 How Does It Work?

The Frankel appliance works in both the antero-posterior and transverse dimensions and is mainly used in mixed dentition class II cases with a lower lip trap. The appliance works in the following way:

- The buccal acrylic shields hold the cheeks away from the teeth, eliminating cheek pressure. This allows for stretching of the periosteum, creating expansion in the transverse dimension.

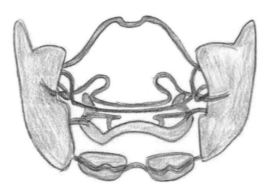

Figure 27.8 Frankel appliance.

- By eliminating any lip interference, the appliance allows forward posturing of the mandible, correcting the antero-posterior dimension.
- By the appliance removing the unfavourable soft tissues, it helps encourage uprighting of the mandibular premolars.

27.8.5.2 Advantages

- Lifetime correction – if the patient cooperates well.
- No surgical correction.
- Movement of tongue is not restricted.
- Less chairside time.
- Used at an early age.
- Removable – does not interfere with patient's oral hygiene.

27.8.5.3 Disadvantages

- Can be difficult to wear.
- Is expensive to make.
- Is troublesome to repair.
- Is rarely used today.
- Is a one-piece appliance.
- Patient is unable to eat and speak with appliance in.

27.8.6 Clip-on Fixed Functional Appliance

The clip-on fixed functional (COFF) appliance (Figure 27.9) is very similar to a Clark's twin block. The only difference between the two is that the COFF appliance is fixed to the teeth and cannot be removed by the patient, essentially making it a fixed twin block that works in the same way. It is a tooth-borne appliance and consists of acrylic bite blocks that are attached to the molar bands. Prior to placement of the appliance, separators are needed before an impression is taken, which allows for space to be created between the contact points to allow placement of the molar bands. The big advantage this appliance has is that it is fixed to the teeth and cannot be removed, making it non-compliance dependent and meaning it is constantly working, allowing for fast and efficient movement.

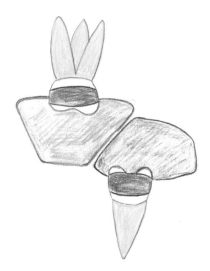

Figure 27.9 Clip-on fixed functional appliance.

27.8.6.1 How Does It Work?

- The appliance consists of acrylic bite blocks and molar bands that are attached together on the upper first permanent molar and lower second premolar.
- The acrylic bite blocks are inclined and help to posture the mandible forward. This is achieved by the lower bite block coming in front of the upper bite block.
- When biting together the bite blocks interlock at 70° to the occlusal surface.

27.8.6.2 Advantages

- Is fixed to the teeth – cannot be removed.
- Works fast and efficiently because it is not removed.
- Patient can eat and speak with it in.
- Is essentially a fixed twin block and works in exactly the same way.
- Is active for 24 hours a day.

27.8.6.3 Disadvantages

- Is hard to keep clean.
- Is difficult to repair.
- Is expensive.
- Frequent appointments are needed prior to fit due to separating contact points for molar bands to be placed and impressions taken for appliance.

27.9 Designing a Functional Appliance

When designing a functional appliance, there are two important factors that need to be considered:

- *Comfort*: ensuring patient comfort is important when designing the appliance, as an uncomfortable appliance will result in the patient not wearing it.
- *Good aesthetics*: functional appliances can be quite bulky, so ensure that the aesthetics of the appliance are reasonable, as poor aesthetics can result in the patient not wearing it.

27.10 Appointments

27.10.1 Records Appointment

After informed consent has been received:

- Records needed: photos, study models, and impressions.
- For functional appliance:
  - Upper and lower alginate impressions.
  - Wax bite needs to be taken when the patient is in maximum protrusion and there is a 6–7 mm separation between the posterior teeth.
- For patients who have a very increased overjet who cannot posture very far forward, another wax bite and set of impressions may need to be taken during the functional appliance treatment so the overjet can be brought back further. However, there are disadvantages of doing this:
  - It requires a new wax bite and impressions, resulting in more time.
  - It is costly.
  - There can be relapse during the time the appliance is being adjusted at the lab.

27.10.2 Fit and Instructions Appointment

- To try the fit and make sure the appliance fits well.
- To adjust retentive components if needed.

- To ensure the patient can insert and remove the appliance themselves.
- To give correct instructions to the patient.
- The appliance can be glued in place for 10–14 days, which prevents the patient from taking it out and gets them used to full-time wear – while this is rarely done, it is an option.

27.10.3   Review Appointments

- Speak to the patient with the appliance in – check for any lisp, signs of wear.
- Check wear – is there an indent on the palate from the appliance, does it show signs of being worn?
- Measure overjet (eventually you want it to be 0 mm).
- Check molar relationship (eventually you want it to be class III).
- Check the fit and adjust if required.
- Reactivate if necessary by the orthodontist if the appliance is modified, for example midline expansion screw or springs.
- Cold cure acrylic can be added or removed at any time, for example acrylic may be added for an upper bite block.

28

Fixed Appliances

28.1 Definition

A fixed appliance is an orthodontic appliance that is fixed to the teeth and cannot be removed by the patient.

28.2 Indications for Fixed Appliances

There are many reasons why fixed appliances may be considered:

- Correction of mild to moderate skeletal discrepancies.
- Intrusion/extrusion of the teeth.
- Correction of rotations.
- Overbite reduction by incisor intrusion.
- Multiple tooth movements in one arch.
- Closure of extraction spaces or spaces due to hypodontia.
- Improve psychological well-being.

28.3 Advantages and Disadvantages

There are many advantages and disadvantages that fixed appliances have over other types of appliances within orthodontics.

Advantages:

- Three-dimensional control of tooth movement.
- Achievement of bodily movement.
- Complex malocclusions can be treated.
- Controlled space closure possible.
- Multiple tooth movements.
- Can be used in both arches.
- Simple to correct rotations.
- Not dependent on compliance.

Textbook for Orthodontic Therapists, First Edition. Ceri Davies.
© 2020 John Wiley & Sons Ltd. Published 2020 by John Wiley & Sons Ltd.

- Intrusion/extrusion of teeth.
- Overbite reduction by incisor intrusion.
- Improve psychological well-being.

  Disadvantages:

- High anchorage requirements.
- Oral hygiene (OH) can become a problem.
- Increased chairside time.
- Require extensive training to manage.
- Gingivitis/periodontitis due to poor OH during treatment.
- Caries due to poor OH during treatment.
- Decalcification.
- Temporomandibular dysfunction (TMD) can become worse or no better.
- Ulceration due to trauma on mucosa.
- Appliance breakages.
- Root resorption.
- Loss of vitality.
- Not very aesthetically pleasing.

28.4   Tooth Movement Achieved with Fixed Appliances

Different types of movement can be achieved with fixed appliances:

- Tipping
- Bodily movement
- Torque
- Extrusion
- Intrusion
- Rotation.

28.5   Mode of Action

The mode of action refers to the forces that are applied to the teeth during fixed appliance treatment. To achieve tooth movement, the force applied must reach the tooth's centre of resistance. These two actions are the moment and the force couple.

$$\text{Moment} = \text{Magnitude of force applied to tooth} \times \text{Perpendicular distance between point of application and centre of resistance}$$

This achieves rotational movement only, although there can be tipping too. Movement is achieved when the line of force that is created does not pass through the centre of resistance. Due to this, the force will translate and rotate the tooth around its centre of resistance.

For example, a palatally displaced lateral with a button bonded labially with chain elastic engaged from the button to the archwire to help bring the tooth anteriorly.

$$\text{Force couple} = \text{Magnitude of forces applied to tooth} \times \text{Distance between them}$$

Two equal and opposite forces produce a force couple, which acts to cause rotation, inclination of the teeth, and torque. This achieves pure rotation around the tooth's centre of resistance. No translation is achieved.

However, force moments and couples do work together to produce bodily movement. When the archwire is engaged into the bracket slot, the force couple created is used to control the tipping that is caused by the force moment. This achieves bodily tooth movement.

28.6 Components of Fixed Appliances

Fixed appliances are made up of four components:

- Bands
- Brackets
- Archwires
- Auxiliaries.

28.6.1 Bands

28.6.1.1 What Are Bands?
Bands are stainless-steel rings, which are placed around the entire crown of a tooth, leaving only the occlusal surface free.

28.6.1.2 Where Are Bands Used?
Bands can be used on molars or premolars.

28.6.1.3 When Can Bands Be Used?
- Bands are used in fixed appliances.
- They are used when failure of a bonded attachment keeps occurring, especially on crowns.
- They are used for headgear, transpalatal arches (TPA), TPA with Nance, rapid maxillary expansion (RME), quadhelix, and lingual arches.
- Bands can have a lingual/palatal attachment which can be soldered or welded on when required.

28.6.1.4 Why Are Bands Used?
- Molars are generally banded because restricted access can make moisture control and accurate positioning for bonding more difficult.
- In fixed appliances some clinicians may prefer to band molars instead of using a buccal tube or because of the large restorations and lack of enamel present, making it difficult to bond the surface.
- Headgear involves banding molars as the extra-oral force will increase the chance of bond failure and the risk of injury to the patient.
- RME, TPA, TPA with Nance, lingual arch, and quadhelix all require molar bands. These are used in conjunction, as the components for each appliance can be soldered or welded onto the lingual/palatal surface of the band.
- Bands are required when brackets cannot be bonded onto:
  - Amalgam
  - Amelogenesis (poor enamel)

– Porcelain
– Fluorosis – a condition caused by overexposure to fluoride during the first eight years of life.

28.6.1.5 How Are Bands Placed/Bonded?

- Prior to bond placement the adjacent tooth contacts are to be separated.
- Separation of contact points involves placing a separation elastic, metal separating spring, or brass wire between the contact points using separating pliers or floss.
- Once enough room is made (after two to seven days), separation elastic is removed prior to band placement if they have not fallen out on their own.
- The appropriate band size is selected. It must sit flush around the tooth to prevent it from coming loose during treatment.
- Glass ionomer cement (GIC) is then used to cement the band in place. After placing the cement around all four sides of the band, it is secured in place using finger pressure. Then the patient is asked to bite down on a bite stick, which seats the band into the correct position. A band seater is then used which will help to make sure that the edges of the band are flush with the tooth mesially and distally.
- GIC is used due to it being:
  - Fluoride releasing
  - Adherent to enamel
  - Sets when in contact with saliva
  - Mixed on a cold slab.
- When placing a band it is important to ensure that the tooth surface is dry and that all excess glue is removed before it sets from the occlusal, gingival, mesial, and distal surfaces of the tooth.
- The indent on the molar tube is always placed on the buccal surface.

28.6.1.6 Advantages of Bands

- There is less chance of them debonding compared to a buccal tube bracket.
- They have increased stability.
- They provide an additional attachment for headgear, TPA, TPA with Nance, and lingual arch on the palatal and buccal sides of the band.

28.6.1.7 Disadvantages of Bands

- Separation is needed prior to bonding to ensure the band can fully fit around the tooth.
- They are less aesthetic than brackets.
- They can irritate the gingiva.
- They are slower to bond than brackets.
- More appointments are needed due to separation and then bonding of the band.
- Increased cost.
- Gaps can be present after debonding.

28.6.1.8 Cementing Bands

There are many types of cements that can be used for cementing bands into place, such as:

- GIC
- Band-Lok® (Reliance Orthodontic Products, Itasca, IL, USA)
- Poly-F® Plus (Dentsply Sirona, York, PA, USA)
- Zinc phosphate.

28.6.1.9   Failure Rate of Bands
The failure rate is 5%.

28.6.2   Brackets

28.6.2.1   What Is a Bracket?
Brackets are attachments bonded onto the crown of a tooth in fixed appliances. They help spread and control the forces that are applied from the archwire and auxiliaries.

28.6.2.2   Where Are Brackets Used?
Brackets are bonded onto the enamel surface of the crown of the tooth. Depending on what appliance is used, brackets can either be bonded onto the labial surface with buccal fixed appliances or on the palatal/lingual surface with lingual appliances.

28.6.2.3   When Are Brackets Used?
Brackets are used throughout fixed appliance treatment.

28.6.2.4   Types of Bracket
There are three different types of brackets that can be used with different fixed appliances: conventional edgewise, ribbonwise, and self-ligating brackets.

28.6.2.4.1   *Conventional Edgewise Brackets*
These brackets use a wire that is thicker horizontally and that fits in the bracket slot.

- Standard edgewise appliance: non-prescription.
- Preadjusted edgewise appliance: prescription in bracket.
- Tip edge: prescription in bracket.

There are two edgewise bracket slot sizes (Figure 28.1):

- 0.018 in.
- 0.022 in.

Characteristics:

- These brackets are fabricated with a single archwire channel and four tie wings.
- They have a reduced interbracket span.
- The width of the bracket is increased, which produces better control of tooth rotations and root position.
- Ligation of the archwire to the bracket slot is by use of elastomeric modules or short ligature.

Advantages:

- They are used in the standard edgewise (no prescription) and preadjusted edgewise (prescription in brackets) appliances.
- Preadjusted edgewise brackets reduce the chance of wire bending being required.
- These brackets can provide good sliding mechanics.
- They can provide good finishing.

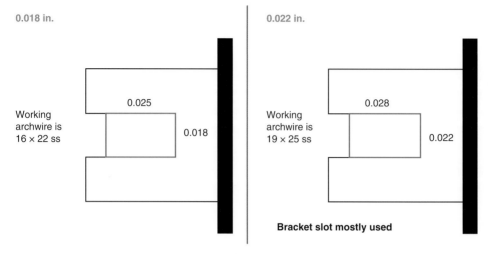

0.018 in.

0.022 in.

Working archwire is 16 × 22 ss

0.025

0.018

Working archwire is 19 × 25 ss

0.028

0.022

Bracket slot mostly used

Figure 28.1 Different bracket slot sizes. ss, stainless steel.

Disadvantages:

- These brackets ignore the biological variation.
- They can produce increased friction, which increases anchorage considerations.
- They can be time consuming when ligating archwire with elastomeric modules and quick ligatures, increasing chairside time.
- Poor OH can arise due to the elastomeric modules.

28.6.2.4.2 Ribbonwise Brackets
These brackets use a wire that is thicker vertically and that fits in the bracket slot.

- Lingual – Incognito® (3M, St Paul, MN, USA)/Harmony® (American Orthodontics, Sheboygan, WI, USA): prescription in bracket.
- Begg: non-prescription bracket.

28.6.2.4.3 Self-ligating Brackets
- Damon® (Ormco, Orange, CA, USA): prescription in bracket; same size as edgewise brackets.

Characteristics:

- These brackets provide low friction.
- Appointment times are reduced due to the ligation built into the bracket.
- Ligation of archwire into the bracket slot is by use of a metal gate or clip.
- Bracket slot can either be passive or active:
  - *Passive*: this bracket has a slide mechanism which is passive and places no active force on the archwire when engaged in the bracket slot.
  - *Active*: an active force is placed on the archwire when engaged in the bracket slot.

Advantages:

- Provide low friction.
- Have more robust ligation.

- Can be more efficient with tooth movement and sliding mechanics.
- Provide enhanced rotational control.
- Reduced chairside adjustment.
- Longer appointment intervals.
- Can achieve full wire engagement.
- Quick and easy to use.
- OH more improved and easier to maintain due to no elastomeric modules.

28.6.2.5 Bracket Materials

There are many different types of bracket materials that can be used, such as:

- Metal
- Stainless steel
- Cobalt-chromium
- Titanium
- Ceramic
- Plastic.

28.6.2.6 Aesthetic Brackets

Two forms of aesthetic brackets are used within orthodontics, which can be made out of:

- *Plastic*: manufactured from polyurethane or polycarbonate reinforced ceramic or fibreglass fillers.
- *Ceramic*: manufactured from aluminium oxide and described as either:
  - Polycrystalline: opaque
  - Monocrystalline: clear.

28.6.2.6.1 Ceramic Brackets

These brackets were introduced in the 1980s and are very popular today. There are many advantages to them: not only are they aesthetically pleasing for patients because of their colour stability, but they provide higher strength and are more resistant than metal brackets to wear and deformation. They also have disadvantages, however. Ceramic brackets provide low friction toughness, which can lead to high bracket breakage. Due to the ceramic being a hard material, this can lead to enamel damage and wear. Damage can occur during the debonding of brackets due to the high bond strength, and enamel wear can occur on opposing teeth, most commonly on the lower incisors in increased overbite cases. Greater friction also occurs with ceramic brackets when the archwire is engaged in the bracket slot; however, to overcome this some ceramic brackets have a metal slot incorporated to reduce friction.

Advantages:

- Good aesthetics.
- Popular with patients.
- Better than plastic.

Disadvantages:

- Can be brittle and fracture.
- Are extremely hard and can cause wear in the opposing arch.
- Give an increased risk of enamel fracture at debonding.

- Increase friction – some brackets now have a metal slot to reduce friction.
- Are expensive.
- Can result in poor positioning due to no jigs or dot.
- Can have poor tie wings, making it difficult to put auxiliaries on.

28.6.2.7 Bracket Manufacturing

Manufacturing of brackets can be done in two ways, which are different and can influence when brackets are debonded. The two ways are:

- *Spot welded*: where the base and body of the brackets are made separately, then stuck together. These are cheaper brackets and the base and body of the bracket can debond away from each other.
- *Injection moulded*: where the base and body of the bracket are injection moulded together in a jig. These brackets are more expensive, but have less chance of debonding during treatment.

With spot-welded brackets, if the base of the bracket remains on the tooth surface, a fast hand-piece can be used to remove the base. Only orthodontists can do this.

28.6.2.8 Bonding Brackets

There are two ways in which brackets can be bonded onto a tooth surface:

- *Direct bonding*: the brackets are placed individually.
- *Indirect bonding*: the brackets are placed on study models in the lab and then transferred to the teeth using a positioning tray.

Once brackets are placed by either the direct or indirect approach, a mechanical and chemical bond is used to achieve adhesion to the tooth surface:

- *Mechanical bond*: this is the interlocking of the molecules. Phosphoric acid (etch) is applied to the tooth surface; once washed and dried it leaves exposed crystalline structures within the enamel. These pitted areas will allow the bond to flow in between these contact points to allow for mechanical bond. This is increased with the mesh base found on the back of the brackets.
- *Chemical bond*: this comes from the composite and primer, which allows for polymerization. That is the process by which two molecules join together, sharing anatomical structures.

Brackets are bonded to the teeth by use of the acid etch technique or self-etch primer, with many modern composites in use today. To assist with bonding, each bracket has a mesh base (Figure 28.2) which helps to achieve mechanical interlock (the mechanical bond described above). The mesh base helps due to the roughened area it provides, allowing for improvement of bond strength against the etched enamel tooth surface. The base is also curved in both the horizontal and vertical planes, which helps bracket location and seating of the bracket on the crown of the tooth.

28.6.2.9 Bracket Orientation

Due to the inbuilt features within each bracket, it is important that the bracket is positioned on the tooth in the correct position. The bracket must be placed in the centre of the clinical crown in relation to where the horizontal and vertical planes meet. However, this can change in some circumstances. For example, if intrusion of a tooth is required, the bracket may be positioned more incisally; whereas for extrusion, the bracket may be positioned more gingivally. Incorrect positioning can result in incorrect tooth positioning.

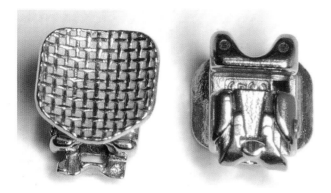

Figure 28.2 Mesh base on the back of a Damon Mx bracket.

28.6.2.10 Bracket Rules

There are many different rules that apply to brackets when bonding them onto the clinical crown. These rules only apply in certain cases and are not considered for every patient. Example are:

- Inverting an upper canine bracket torques the root palatally.
  - Turning the bracket upside down on canine teeth may be considered in a hypodontia case where upper laterals are missing.
  - The reason this is considered is because lateral incisor roots are more inclined palatally and when a canine is camouflaging lateral incisors, inverting the bracket will help torque the root of the canine more palatally.
- Inverting a lateral incisor bracket torques root labially.
  - Turning the bracket upside down on a lateral incisor helps bring the root labially, starting to correct the position from the beginning of treatment.
  - This is considered in cases where laterals are positioned very palatally.
- Swapping lower canine brackets (L for R and R for L) prevents forward tip of the canines.
  - This is considered in class III cases and can be very useful.
  - Swapping these brackets over helps prevent forward tip of the lower canines, preventing the lower anterior teeth from proclining forward, which can result in the patient looking more class III.
- Inverting lower incisor brackets in MBT tilts the incisors forwards.
  - Turning the lower incisor brackets upside down in the MBT system helps tilt the lower incisors forwards. This changes the torque prescription in the bracket, allowing these teeth to procline.
  - This is considered in severe class II cases, as it will help to reduce the increased overjet.

Figure 28.3 gives the tip and torque values within the MBT bracket prescription.

28.6.3 Archwires

28.6.3.1 What Are Archwires?

Archwires help to generate biomechanical forces, which are distributed through the brackets to achieve tooth movement.

UPPER

	1	2	3	4	5	6	7
Tip	4	8	8	0	0	0	0
Torque	17	10	−7	−7	−7	−14	−14
Tooth	**1**	**2**	**3**	**4**	**5**	**6**	**7**
Tip	0	0	3	2	2	0	0
Torque	−6	−6	−6	−12	−17	−20	−10

LOWER

Figure 28.3 MBT bracket prescription values.

28.6.3.2 What Are Archwires Used For?

Archwires have many functions within orthodontic treatment, such as:

- *Force*: they provide the force to move the teeth.
- *Track*: they act as a track which the teeth move along.
- *Pattern*: they provide a pattern for the shape of the arch.
- *Engagement*: they exert forces by being engaged in the bracket slot.

28.6.3.3 What Are Archwires Used?

Archwires are used throughout the different stages of treatment:

- Levelling and alignment (in/out, up/down), to correct crossbites and rotations.
- Overbite reduction.
- Overjet reduction.
- Space closure.
- Finishing and detailing.
- Retention.

28.6.3.4 Archwire Properties

Each archwire has physical properties, but not all properties can be found in one archwire. However, the ideal physical properties are dependent on the stage of treatment. As there is no archwire that offers all of these physical properties, a sequence of archwires is needed for fixed appliance treatment to help achieve tooth movement. Each archwire sequence will depend on the clinician's personal choice.

The seven main physical properties found in archwires are:

- *Springback*: when the wire returns to its original shape after a force is applied.
- *Stiffness*: the amount of force required to deflect or bend an archwire.
- *Formability*: when the wire is able to be bent into the desired shape.
- *Resilience*: the energy stored in the wire to move teeth when it is deformed.
- *Biocompatibility*: non-allergenic archwire.
- *Joinability*: whether the material can be soldered or welded for auxiliaries.
- *Frictional characteristics*: low surface friction is needed for optimum tooth movement.

Which properties are needed at which stage of treatment?

- Initial stages of treatment for tooth alignment and de-rotation:
  - Large springback
  - Low stiffness
  - High stored energy – resilience
  - Biocompatibility
  - Low surface friction – frictional characteristics.
- Mid-treatment stage for overbite reduction and sliding of teeth along archwire:
  - High stiffness
  - Low stored energy – resilience
  - Biocompatibility
  - Low surface friction – frictional characteristics
  - Good joinability.
- Mid-treatment stage for space closure to reduce an overjet:
  - High stiffness
  - Low stored energy – resilience
  - Biocompatibility
  - Low surface friction – frictional characteristics
  - Good joinability.

28.6.3.5 Archwire Materials

Archwires come from the fabrication of metal alloys. Metal alloys consist of two or more elements, which are combined by mixing in a molten state. Changing the elements in the alloy can change the properties of the metal alloys. Metal alloys offer all different physical properties, which is why we have a sequence of archwires for the different stages of treatment. The alloys found within archwires are known to be strong and corrosion resistant. The metal alloys used for archwire are as follows:

- Stainless steel
- Nickel titanium (NiTi, CuNiti, HANT)
- Beta titanium (TMA)
- Cobalt-chromium.

28.6.3.5.1 *Stainless Steel*

Stainless steel is an alloy of iron, nickel, and chromium and became a very popular material to use for orthodontic archwires in the 1950s. Stainless-steel archwires are considered when more force and stiffness are needed. This is due to the material being stiffer. However, the disadvantage of this is that the archwire does not deflect as much, making it produce a stronger force, resulting in patient discomfort. Due to this discomfort, stainless-steel archwires only provide pressure and movement for a short period of time.

This material can be made flexible by twisting several very thin strands of 0.0075 in. wire to give a 0.16 in. multistrand archwire that is a similar size to a nickel titanium archwire. These archwires are considered for use when bends within the archwire are needed. This is because they take a permanent set when bent and are easy to adjust when bends and curves are to be placed.

The advantages of this type of material in archwires are that it is low cost, has excellent formability and has good mechanical properties. Stainless-steel archwires can be soldered or welded and can have hooks soldered on. Another alternative is having loops placed within the archwire. This increases the span of wire between the brackets and therefore will increase the flexibility; however, this is only useful when a rigid archwire is desirable in other areas within the arch. For space closure, stainless-steel archwires are considered due to good sliding mechanics being achieved and the low friction that is produced when brackets move along the archwire. The material can be softened by annealing (heating) the archwire.

28.6.3.5.2 Nickel Titanium
NiTi archwires have two properties:

- *Thermal shape memory*: this property returns the archwire to its original shape, especially if there is an increase in temperature, for example the patient drinking a cup of tea.
- *Superelasticity*: this property allows the wire to be deflected much further than other materials and still return to its original shape.

These archwires are very well known for their high flexibility and provide a light (gentle) continuous force. In the levelling and aligning stages of treatment, they are used because, when they are cooled, they are more flexible. This allows the wire to be deflected, which makes it easier for the wire to be inserted into the mouth and tied into displaced teeth. Appointment intervals can be made longer with these archwires, as movement can occur over a long period of time, from weeks and even up to months.

The disadvantages of these archwires are that they have a high surface roughness, which increases friction, and they become stiffer when warmed up in the mouth. Cool foods such as ice cream will help patients when teeth are tender, as this will cool the archwire and relieve any discomfort they may be experiencing.

There are many other different types of nickel titanium archwires, such as:

- Nitinol:
  - The Naval Ordnance Laboratory in the USA began making nitinol archwires in the early 1960s. They contain the same properties as NiTi archwires; that is, thermal memory and superelasticity. Nitinol provides the same low continuous force and has good flexibility, making it easy to tie into displaced teeth. Nitinol archwires are martensitic stabilised, meaning they are soft at room temperature until they are inserted into the mouth, but become stiffer when working.
- Heat-activated nickel titanium (HANT):
  - HANT archwires are more flexible when chilled and are thermally active once in the mouth. They start off being martensitic active, then turn into austenitic active in the mouth.
- Copper nickel titanium (CuNiTi):
  - CuNiTi archwires are very popular today. They are mainly used at the initial stage of treatment, because they can be deflected much further and still return to their original shape. The copper is the main component that makes the archwire more resistant (harder) to permanent deformation; as the amount of copper is increased, it also increases the sensitivity of the archwire to temperature. When the archwire is out of the mouth it is cool or 'dead soft', making it more flexible and easier to insert into the patient's mouth, whereas when it is warm it becomes active, which makes it stiffer. Due to this heat activation, CuNiTi archwires start off as martensitic active then turn to austenitic once in the mouth. The archwire has three temperature variants, which change the wire structure:

- o 27° – Useful for mouth breathers.
- o 35° – Activated at normal body temperature.
- o 40° – Activated after hot drinks.
- Superelastic NiTi:
  - This archwire material has good superelasticity and thermal memory properties within it. It has good flexibility, but only if it is deflected by more than 3 mm, as it starts off being austenitic active, then turns to martensitic. A low continuous force is achieved with this archwire.

All nickel titanium archwires hold austenitic and martensitic active properties:

- *Austenitic active*: an austenitic NiTi wire can change from the stiffer phase to a martensitic (more flexible) phase if deflected more than 3 mm. As the teeth move the deflection decreases; the wire becomes stiffer as the proportion of austenite increases.
  - Austenitic active archwires: superelastic, NiTi.
- *Martensitic active*: these wires are soft at room temperature (martensitic phase), and change from martensitic to austenitic at mouth temperature. This is a flexible archwire before it is inserted into the mouth.
  - Martensitic active archwires: nitinol, HANT or CuNiTi.
  - HANT and CuNiTi are martensitic active at rest, then turn to austenitic at mouth temperature.

28.6.3.5.3   Titanium Molybdenum Alloy

TMA stands for titanium molybdenum alloy or beta titanium and is an alloy of titanium 80%, molybdenum 10%, and zirconium 6%. This archwire material contains no nickel and is good for patients who have a nickel allergy. It is mainly used as a transitional wire and for any final detailing in the finishing stage of treatment. This is another alternative to using a stainless-steel wire, as the wire also takes a permanent set when bent and has medium-range stiffness, with elasticity 40% that of stainless steel. The only disadvantage is that it is expensive. The advantage of using this archwire is that it has high springback and produces a lower force than a stainless-steel archwire. Welding of the material can be achieved if other wires and auxiliaries need to be attached to the archwire, such as hooks for elastic wear.

28.6.3.5.4   Cobalt-Chromium

This archwire material is commercially marketed as Elgiloy® (Elgiloy Speciality Metals, Sycamore, IL, USA). It has greater formability than and similar stiffness to stainless steel; however, it does produce greater friction. This material is frequently used for the construction of auxiliaries such as an intrusion arch or quadhelix. One advantage is that heat treating in the laboratory can harden this archwire material.

28.6.3.6   Archwire Archforms

All archwires come in different archforms. This is to help maintain the patient's lower inter-canine, inter-molar and lower labial section widths. When choosing archforms it is important to maintain as close to the patient's original form as possible, as this will minimise relapse. Archforms come in many shapes, including ovoid, square and tapered (Figure 28.4).

To ensure the correct archform is chosen for the patient, templates are available to assess the patient's lower arch shape. For example, a euro arch form or wax bite of the patient's lower arch

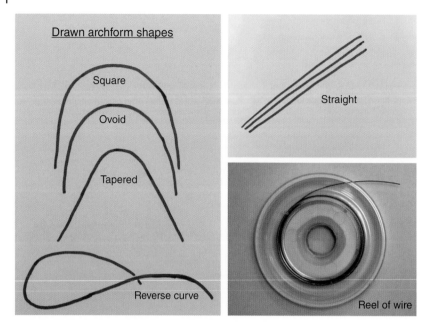

Figure 28.4 Different archforms used in fixed appliances.

can be taken. This will show the indentations of the brackets. When the lower archform has been determined, the upper archwire should coordinate 3 mm further buccally to the lower arch.

28.6.3.7 Archwire Shapes and Sizes

Archwires come in different shapes and sizes for fixed appliance treatment. The shapes that archwires can come in are:

- Round:
  - Round archwires (Figure 28.5) are used in the initial and first middle stages of treatment. When used in the middle stages of treatment they are referred to as 'working archwires'.
  - Round archwires are a solid length of wire and it is important for them to have good flexibility, especially in the first, initial stage (levelling and aligning), as the flexibility will make it easier for the archwire to be tied into displaced teeth.
  - These archwires will only produce a tipping movement to the teeth, which is what is required in the first stage of treatment, as this will help the teeth to level and align.
  - As well as being good for flexibility, archwires must have a medium stiffness too, but should only provide a gentle light force.
  - Round wires can be bent up, down, in, or out in order to move individual teeth, which make it easier at the beginning of treatment for the wire to be tied into displaced teeth.
- Rectangular and square:
  - Rectangular/square archwires (Figures 28.6 and 28.7) are used in the second middle and final stages of treatment. They are a solid length of wire and are stiffer than round archwires.
  - When these archwires are used, the levelling and aligning of the crowns of the teeth should be complete and torque of the roots is then needed.

- Unlike round wires, rectangular wires fill more of the bracket slot and provide more control to torque the roots of the teeth.
- The difference with rectangular wires is that they are even thicker in the mesio-distal direction that the occlusal-gingival direction.
- Multistranded
  - Multistranded round and rectangular wires are also available and can come in many different materials, such as stainless steel, NiTi, CuNiTi, or TMA.
- Solid.

Wire of any material can be round, square, rectangular, or multistranded. The cross-section determines what kind of force the wire is going to produce.

Each archwire also comes in different sizes, with single figures being the round archwires and double figures being the rectangular/square archwires. Sizes of archwires can range from 0.014 in. to 0.019 in. × 0.025 in., with many intermediate sizes available.

The diameter of the wire helps to determine the size of the wire and the cross-section is what is measured when referring to the size of the archwire (Figure 28.8). The diameter is not just used for size, but allows more freedom within the bracket slot to enable the wire to tip the teeth.

The diameter also helps determine the size of the archwire in a square or rectangular archwire. The cross-section on these archwires is measured the same way a round archwire is. Measuring the cross-section will indicate the size of the archwire. The area of the cross-section is the length times the height (Figure 28.9).

28.6.3.8 Degree of Slop

The degree of slop is a term used for the amount of play that is found between the archwire and the bracket on engagement. The amount of slop within the bracket can be different at any time because of the difference between the dimensions of the archwire and the bracket slot itself:

- Round wires: more slop is found due to less friction within the bracket slot.
- Rectangular wires: less slop is found due to more friction within the bracket slot and torqueing of the roots of the teeth. With a rectangular archwire, however, 10° of slop is still found.

28.6.3.9 Archwire Sequence

The choice of archwires depends on the stage of treatment it is being used in and the properties needed to achieve the tooth movements that are required. The next archwire cannot be placed until the previous archwire has been engaged to all the teeth. There is no certain sequence that clinicians have to go by; every clinician is different and has their own preferred archwire sequence.

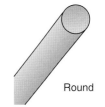

Figure 28.5 Round archwire.

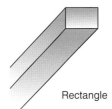

Figure 28.6 Rectangular archwire.

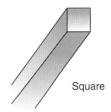

Figure 28.7 Square archwire.

Figure 28.8 How the diameter (size) of the wire is measured: round archwire.

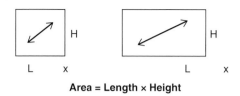

Area = Length × Height

Figure 28.9 How the diameter (size) of the wire is measured: square and rectangular archwire.

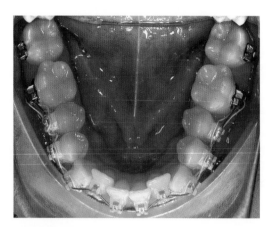

Figure 28.10 Lower occlusal view after bonding of lower fixed appliance.

28.6.3.9.1 Initial Stage of Treatment

Archwires in this stage of treatment are used to correct levelling and aligning, derotation of teeth, and correction of crossbites. These movements are all corrected by tipping the teeth. Round flexible archwires are needed to provide a gentle continuous force that is flexible enough to engage the brackets on the misaligned teeth (Figure 28.10).

NiTi and CuNiTi are the round flexible archwires that are considered.

Sizes used in this stage of treatment:

- 0.012 in., considered in very crowded cases
- 0.013 in., considered in very crowded cases
- 0.014 in.
- 0.016 in., considered if unable to engage 0.018 in.
- 0.018 in.

28.6.3.9.2 First Middle Stage of Treatment

Round wires can be considered for this stage for overbite reduction, overjet reduction, and space closure. Wires with increased stiffness and good sliding mechanics are required (Figure 28.11). The increased stiffness provides a stronger force, with low friction making the brackets move along the archwire easily. These archwires are known as 'working wires'.

Sizes used in this stage of treatment:

- Overbite reduction:
  - Round stainless-steel archwire, 0.016, 0.018, or 0.020 in.
  - Round 0.018 in. reverse-curve (rc) stainless-steel or NiTi archwire – this archwire will extrude the molars and intrude the incisors.

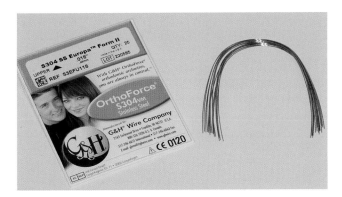

Figure 28.11   Stainless-steel archwires.

- The patient can then go from rc to 16×16, then 17×25 rc to level and finish the curve of Spee if necessary.
  - Or 14×25, 18×25, then 17×25 rc NiTi to level the curve of Spee if necessary.
- Overjet reduction and space closure:
  - 0.016, 0.018, or 0.020 in. round stainless-steel wires.
  - Elastics can be started at this stage – classes II, III.

Adjustment appointments can vary for different appliances. Depending on what system is used, some patients' archwire changes can vary from anything between 4 and 6 and up to 12–14 weeks.

28.6.3.9.3   Second Middle Stage of Treatment
Rectangular archwires are used for this stage to help finish the overbite and overjet reduction, finish space closure, and start the initial torque to the teeth.

The archwires used for this are NiTi and CuNiTi. Sizes used in this stage of treatment:

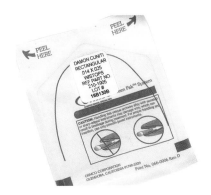

Figure 28.12   Damon copper nickel titanium rectangular archwire, 0.14×0.25 in.

- 16×16 heat-activated NiTi and CuNiTi
- 14×25 CuNiTi/NiTi (Figure 28.12)
- 16 × 25 CuNiTi/NiTi
- 17 × 25 CuNiTi/NiTi
- 18×25 CuNiTi/NiTi
- 17×25 rc NiTi (Figure 28.13), additional wire if needed to achieve a flat curve of Spee.

Not all these archwires are used in this stage; it all depends on what type of sequence the clinician prefers. If space closure is still needed, a stainless-steel archwire will be preferred where chain elastic and elastics can be used, for example a 16×22 stainless-steel archwire may be considered.

Adjustment appointments can vary for different appliances. Depending on what system is used, some

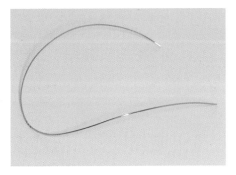

Figure 28.13   Reverse-curve archwire.

patients' archwire changes can vary from anything between 4 and 6 and up to 12–14 weeks. For finishing space closure, patients can be seen at 6–8 weeks for frequent changing of the chain elastic.

28.6.3.9.4 Final Stage of Treatment

Rectangular archwires are used in this stage for final detailing of tooth positions, final torque, and settling down of the occlusion. Stainless-steel or TMA rectangular archwires are considered for this because they take a permanent set when bends are placed in them for final tooth detailing.

The archwires used in this stage are usually flexible, which will allow for final adjustments such as wire bending.

Sizes used in this stage of treatment:

- 19×25 stainless steel
- 19×25 TMA (Figure 28.14)
- 21 × 25 TMA.

Adjustment appointments can vary for different appliances. Depending on what system is used, archwires can be left in situ for around 8–12 weeks. However, 4 weeks may be considered if bends are placed to allow the wire to work.

Before changing the patient's archwire, it is important to know whether the current archwire is still active or passive. If the archwire is active, it means it is still working and you can see this, as the archwire will not move between the bracket slots and will not slide from side to side. However, for a passive archwire this means the job has been done and the archwire can move and shift from side to side. This is a good indication of when the next archwire is ready for engagement.

28.6.4 Auxiliaries

28.6.5 What Are Auxiliaries?

Auxiliaries are additional components that are used on fixed appliances. They are categorised into two groups:

- Metal auxiliaries:
  - Metal ligatures (Figure 28.15) – long or short (can be aesthetic)
  - Coil spring (Figure 28.16) – stainless steel or NiTi
    - Open active coil helps to make spaces
    - Closed passive coil helps to maintain spaces

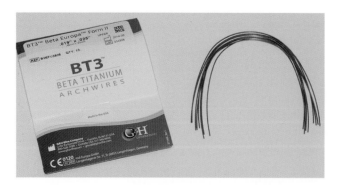

Figure 28.14 Beta titanium archwires.

Metal ligatures

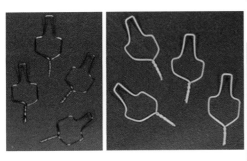

Short:
- Also known as quick ligatures
- Used to ligate wire into bracket slot especially on conventional appliances – can be used on self-ligating brackets when wire cannot be engaged into bracket slot
- More rigid and firm

Can be aesthetic – white ligatures

Long:
- Used as a laceback 3-6 (figure of 8) – helps to prevent teeth tipping mesially, preventing gaps appearing and to start bring canines back into an extraction space
- Used as an undertie 3-3, 6-6, or 7-7 (figure of 8), used as an anchor unit in elastic traction, maintain position of teeth and to prevent gaps appearing
- Used to extrude canines – exposed canine. Long ligature is activated to help bring impacted tooth or dispalced teeth to the alignment

Can be aesthetic – white ligatures

Figure 28.15 Short and long metal ligatures.

Coil spring
- Constructed from SS or NiTi
- Two types: open and closed

Open:
- Active spring
- Used for opening spaces

Closed:
- Passive spring
- Used for maintaining space

Kobayashi hooks

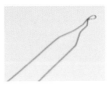

Short:
- Hook can be placed around bracket by Mathieu pliers and tightened around for elastic wear

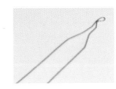

Long:
- Can be used as a hook and undertie

Can be aesthetic too – white ligatures

Figure 28.16 Coil spring and Kobayashi hooks. NiTi, nickel titanium; SS, stainless steel.

- Kobayashi hooks (Figure 28.16) – long or short
- Crimpable hooks (Figure 28.17)
- Crimpable stops (Figure 28.17) – two different types, slide on and envelope
- Buttons (Figure 28.18) – base shape

Crimpable hooks

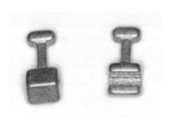

- Hooks placed onto rectangular wires only for elastic wear

- These hooks are known as crimpable hooks because they are squeezed onto wire

Crimpable stops

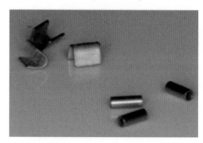

Two types:

- Slide on = these stops slide onto the archwire
- Crimpable = also known as envelope stoppers, these stops are placed and squeezed onto the wire by Weingart pliers. They also help open space by reactivating coil springs by being placed next to the coil spring. These stoppers are used to stop the archwire from shifting in the patient's mouth

Figure 28.17 Crimpable hooks and stops.

**Buttons
Base shape**

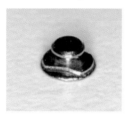

- Constructed in stainless steel. Can be used for:
- Exposed canines – button used to help extrude tooth via metal ligature or chain elastic to bring the tooth into alignment
- Displaced teeth – button placed on displaced tooth with help to bring this tooth to alignment via metal ligature by activation or chain elastic. Activated until bracket can be placed
- Derotated teeth – buttons can be placed for derotation via metal ligature on activation or chain elastic to help rotate tooth to correct position – buttons can be placed palatally/lingually/labially
- Elastic traction – used for crossbite elastics placed on palatal surface to help correct crossbites

Eyelets

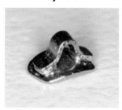

- Constructed in stainless steel. Can be used for:
- Displaced teeth – bonded onto these teeth which are severely crowded for early traction which are unable to be engaged to the wire – these are activated by use of a metal ligature to activate tooth to bring it to alignment with open coil spring to make room for the tooth – open space
- Exposed teeth – used to extrude these teeth when partially erupted with metal ligature on activation to bring this tooth to alignment
- Partially erupted teeth – used on partially erupted teeth to engage to the archwire to extrude them more until a bracket can be placed on the tooth surface to correct the alignment of the tooth itself

Figure 28.18 Buttons and eyelets.

- Eyelets (Figure 28.18)
- Drop-in hooks (Figure 28.19)
- Rotation springs
- Gold chain (Figure 28.19)

Drop in hooks

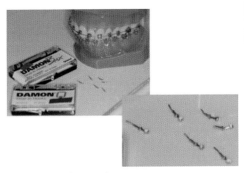

- Used for elastic wear
- Hooks placed into the bracket slot
- Used on self-ligating brackets
- Different Types:
  - Q
  - Mx
  - Insignia

Gold chain

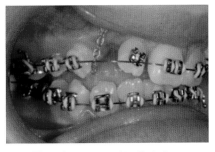

- Placed on exposed teeth during surgical exposure
- Gold chain helps the clinician place metal ligatures through links of chain to help activate this tooth to extrude it through the gum
- At each activation metal ligature is placed through new link getting closer to the tooth

Figure 28.19 Drop-in hooks used for Damon and gold chain.

NiTi retraction spring

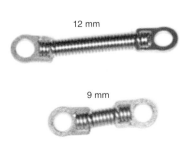

12 mm

9 mm

- Used to close spaces
- Spring attached to retraction hooks on brackets to help close space – retract back
- Used on posted archwires to close space
- Used for intra-arch mechanics
- Come in different sizes – 9 mm or 12 mm
- Activated half a tooth width = 50%

Metal separator

This part sits above the contact point

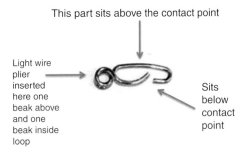

Light wire plier inserted here one beak above and one beak inside loop

Sits below contact point

- Used exactly same way as elastic separators

- Placed by using the light wire pliers

Figure 28.20 Nickel titanium (NiTi) retraction spring and metal separator.

- NiTi retraction springs (Figure 28.20) – different sizes
- Metal separators (Figure 28.20)
- Temporary anchorage devices (TADs; Figure 28.21)
- TPA and TPA with Nance

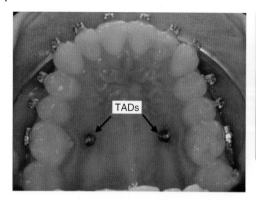
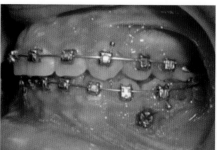
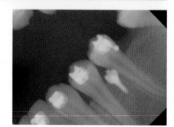

- Screwed into the bone through attached gingiva
- Used to hold teeth or move teeth
- Tooth/teeth attached to TAD directly or indirectly
- Anchorage device

Figure 28.21 Temporary anchorage devices (TADs).

- Lingual arch
- Quadhelix
- RME

- Elastic auxiliaries:
  - Elastomeric modules (Figure 28.22)
  - Elastic bands (Figure 28.23)
  - Intramaxillary elastics (Figures 28.24–28.28)
  - Intra-oral elastics (Figure 28.29)
    - These range in strength (2 oz light, 3 oz medium, 3.5 oz medium heavy, 4.5 oz heavy, and 6 oz extra heavy) and size (1/18, 3/16, ¼, 5/16, 3/8, ½, 5/8, and 3/4 in.)
  - Extra-oral elastics
    - Component of headgear
    - Used instead of a safety module
    - Spring mechanism for pull from facebow to head or neck strap
    - Generally made from latex or polyurethane.
  - Separating modules (Figure 28.30)
  - Rotation wedges (Figure 28.30)
  - Power chain (Figure 28.31) – closed or spaced
  - Power thread (Figure 28.31)
  - Retraction modules (also known as Burman ligs; Figure 28.32)
  - Bumper sleeve (Figure 28.32)
  - Archwire sleeving (tubing)

- Used to hold archwire in bracket slot on conventional appliances
- Placed by using mosquito forceps
- Gently stretched to ease placement

- There are two types:

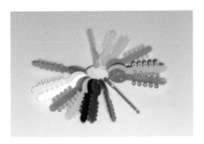

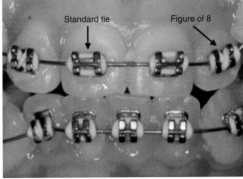

Standard tie   Figure of 8

Standard tie:
Less frictional force on
the archwire

Figure of 8:
Increases frictional force on
the archwire

Figure 28.22 Elastomeric modules.

Elastic bands

Class II

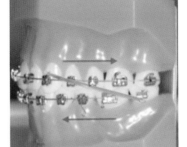

- Usually latex-free elastics
- Used to help achieve tooth movement and correct the malocclusion
- Can be used:
  - ➢ Intra-arch = within single arch
  - ➢ Inter-arch = between the arches
- Different types of elastic wear:

Class I

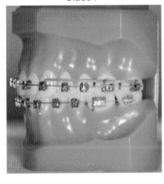

- Intra-arch elastic
- Used for space closure

- These elastics usually attach from the upper canine hook to either the bottom first molar hook or second molar hook
- These elastics help move the upper teeth back and the bottom teeth forward

Figure 28.23 Intermaxillary elastics: elastic bands.

Class III

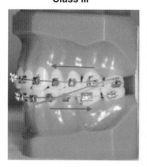

- This elastic starts from the bottom canine and goes to the upper first molar or second molar
- This moves your upper teeth forwards and bottom teeth back
- This is the opposite movement from a class II elastic

Anterior triangle elastics

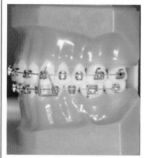

- These elastics usually run from the upper canine hook to the bottom canine and bottom first premolar hooks, forming the shape of a triangle
- This helps in open bite situations where the top front teeth do not touch the bottom front teeth

Class II triangle elastic

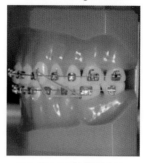

- Like the class II elastic, this elastic starts from the upper canine hook. It also attaches to a bottom bicuspid hook along with the bottom first molar or second molar hook, forming a triangle
- This helps move the upper teeth back and bottom teeth forward and also helps bring the back teet ln together and touching

Figure 28.24 Intermaxillary elastics: class III and triangle elastics.

Class III triangle elastic

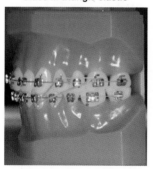

- Like the class III elastic, this elastic starts from the bottom canine hook. It also attaches to a upper bicuspid hook along with the upper first molar or second molar hook, forming a triangle
- This helps move the upper teeth forward and bottom teeth back and also helps bring the· back teeth together and touching

V elastics and Zigzag elastics (finishing elastics)

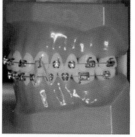

Anterior V elastic

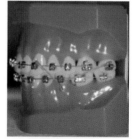

Posterior V elastic

- These elastics attach to three teeth and form the shape of a V
- These elastics help bring teeth together and touching
- They can be used on front teeth or back teeth

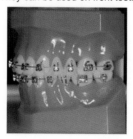

Zigzag elastics

- These elastics help to bring the teeth together during the finishing stages

Figure 28.25 Intermaxillary elastics: class III triangle, V, and zigzag elastics.

Posterior box elastics	Anterior box elastics	Midline elastics

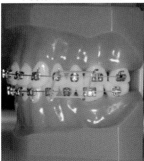

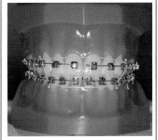

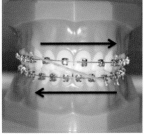

		This elastic can run from the upper canine hook to the bottom canine hook, but it can also be attached to other front teeth. This helps line up the centre of the upper and bottom front teeth
	• This elastic is attached to the anterior teeth in a shape of a box	
• This elastic is attached to four teeth: two on the upper and two on the bottom, forming the shape of a box	• These elastics close down anterior open bites	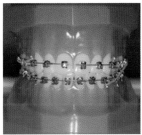
• Can be attached to any configuration of teeth but is most commonly used on the back teeth	**OR**	
	• Class II one side – bring upper teeth on that side posterior and lower teeth anterior	
• This helps to bring the teeth together and touching, closing any posterior open bites	• Class III one side – bring upper teeth anterior and lower teeth posterior	
	All = correction of centreline	

Figure 28.26 Intermaxillary elastics: box and midline elastics.

Crossbite elastics

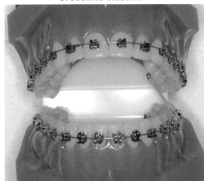

These elastics usually run from the palatal surface of an upper tooth to the buccal surface of a lower tooth to help correct a crossbite (a situation where the upper teeth are inside the bottom teeth)

Lingual crossbite elastics

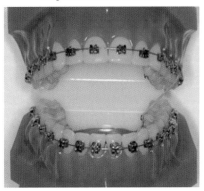

These elastics usually run from the lingual surface of a lower tooth to the buccal surface of an upper tooth to help correct a lingual crossbite (a situation where the lower teeth are further inside the upper teeth than the normal range)

Figure 28.27 Intermaxillary elastics: crossbite elastics.

Class II shudy elastics

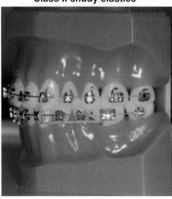

- Combined vertical and AP direction
- Help to increase the overbite and interdigitation of posterior segments:

  - Down and back of upper
  - Forward and up of lower

Class III shudy elastics

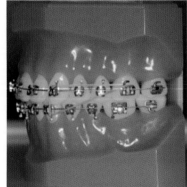

- Combined vertical and AP direction
- Help to increase the overbite and interdigitation of posterior segments:

  - Up and back of lower
  - Forward and down of upper

Figure 28.28 Intermaxillary elastics: Shudy elastics. AP, anterio-posterior.

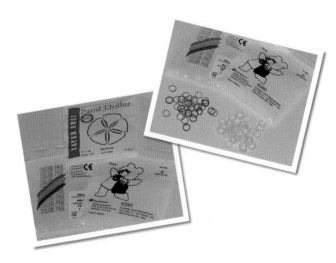

Figure 28.29 Intra-oral elastics.

Separating modules

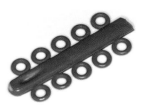

- Used to create space prior to band placement
- Placed into the interproximal areas to make space so the band can sit flush around the tooth
- Placed by separation forceps

Rotation wedges

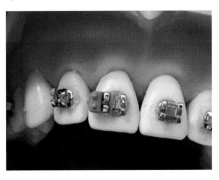

- Rotation wedge attachment is placed over the tie wings of a bracket
- Attachment helps add extra deflection in the wire to help rotate tooth
- They increase force
- Increase spring back of wire – derotation

Figure 28.30 Separating modules and rotation wedges.

Power chain

- Used to close spaces of individual or multiple teeth
- Shift certain teeth to alignment
- Maintain tooth position to prevent any gaps appearing during treatment
- Help to derotate teeth
- Bring displaced teeth to correct alignment
- Two types:

Closed power chain

- Used to close small gaps found between the contact points of teeth

Spaced power chain

- Used to start initial close of large gaps such as diastema before progressing onto the closed power chain

Power thread

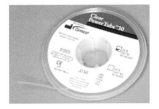

Used on partially erupted and displaced teeth to extrude and bring to correct alignment

Figure 28.31 Power chain and power thread.

Retraction modules (Burnham ligs)

- Made up of a long metal ligature and elastomeric module
- They help close spaces
- Used intra-arch only
- Retraction module placed on metal ligature.
- Metal ligature is twisted with Mathieu pliers and placed on hooks of brackets either end to close spaces

Bumper sleeve

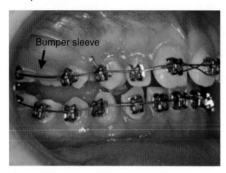

- Soft

- Placed if needed to protect soft tissues adjacent to a wide span of wire

Figure 28.32   Burnham lig and bumper sleeve.

28.6.6   When Do We Use Auxiliaries?

Auxiliaries are used to perform specific tasks in orthodontic tooth movement for the successful use of fixed appliances. They help to generate a force.

28.6.7   Placing Auxiliaries

Orthodontists, orthodontic therapists, and dentists with a special interest in orthodontics can all place auxiliaries onto a fixed appliance.

29

Headgear

29.1 Definition

Headgear is an orthodontic appliance that provides extra-oral anchorage (EOA) and extra-oral traction (EOT) outside of the mouth via attachment of another orthodontic appliance (fixed or removable).

29.2 Extra-Oral Anchorage

EOA is a method used to prevent unwanted tooth movement outside of the mouth:

- It prevents forward movement of molars.
- Force is applied behind the head to hold the anchor teeth back – leading to distalisation of molars.
- Reinforcement of anchorage occurs.

  The magnitude of EOA is 200–250 g of force per side.
  The duration is 10–12 hours a day.

29.3 Extra-Oral Traction

EOT is a method of moving teeth using forces that are outside of the mouth.

- It prevents forward movement of molars.
- Force is applied behind the head to hold the anchor teeth back.
- Achieves tooth movement:
  - Distalisation of molars
  - Extrusion of molars
  - Intrusion of molars
  - Maxillary restraint
  - Reduction in overjet
  - Correction of crossbites

Textbook for Orthodontic Therapists, First Edition. Ceri Davies.
© 2020 John Wiley & Sons Ltd. Published 2020 by John Wiley & Sons Ltd.

- Increase or decrease in lower anterior facial height/Frankfort-mandibular plane angle (LAFH/FMPA)
- Creating space
- Encouraging growth rotations.

Magnitude of EOT is 400–500 g of force per side.
Duration of EOT is 14–16 hours of wear.

29.4 Biomechanics of Headgear

Headgear can achieve the following:

- Distalisation of molars
- Extrusion of molars
- Intrusion of molars
- Maxillary restraint
- Correction of crossbites
- Reduction in overjet
- Creating space
- Increase or decrease of LAFH/FMPA
- Encouraging growth rotations.

29.5 Types of Headgear

There are three different types of pull headgear:

- Cervical (low) pull headgear (Figure 29.1):
  - Achieves:
    - Distalisation and extrusion of molars
    - Increase in the LAFH by extrusion of molars in patients with a low or decreased LAFH.
  - Used on patients presenting with:
    - Skeletal II pattern.
    - Decreased LAFH/FMPA.
    - Deepbite/increased overbite. Extruding the posterior segment in the maxilla encourages a backward growth rotation of the mandible and increase in the MMPA and LAFH furthers buccal extrusion, reducing the deepbite.
    - Forward growth rotation.
    - Force is transmitted below the occlusal plane.
- Combi (straight) pull headgear (Figure 29.2):
  - Achieves distalisation of molars and EOA.
  - Contains both high and low pull.
  - Force is transmitted level with the occlusal plane.
- High pull headgear (Figure 29.3):
  - Achieves:
    - Distalisation of molars
    - Intrusion of molars
    - Maxillary restraint.

Figure 29.1 Cervical low pull headgear.

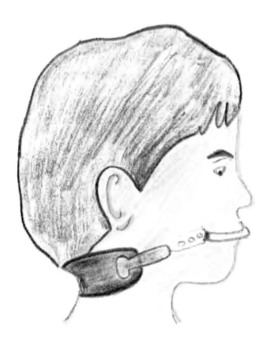

Figure 29.2 Combi straight pull headgear.

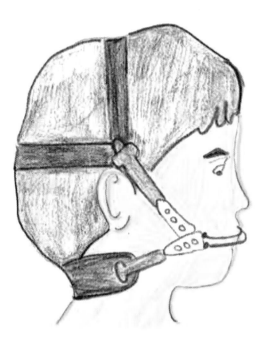

- Used in patients presenting with:
  - ○ Skeletal III pattern.
  - ○ Increased LAFH/FMPA.
  - ○ Anterior overbite (AOB) or decreased overbite. Intruding the posterior segment in the maxilla encourages a forward growth rotation of the mandible and reduction in the MMPA and LAFH furthers buccal intrusion, reducing the AOB.
  - ○ Backward growth rotation.

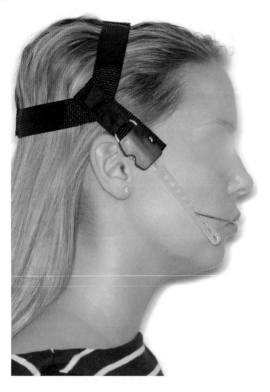

Figure 29.3 High pull headgear.

- Intrusion of molars is desirable for people with an AOB and increased LAFH/FMPA, as doing this reduces the increased LAFH by reducing the AOB.
  - ○ Force is transmitted above the occlusal plane. The centre of resistance is found at the premolar region on the maxilla, which is where the force passes through for maxillary restraint.

29.6   Components of Headgear

The components of headgear are divided into three different sections:

- Ways of attachment to the teeth:
  - Facebow:
    - ○ Removable and functional appliances: a tube is soldered onto the bridge of an Adams clasp where the headgear can slot into (Figure 29.4) or the appliance can have clips over the molar tubes.
    - ○ Fixed appliances: tubes found on molar bands can allow the headgear to slot into them.
  - J hooks:
    - ○ Fixed appliances: these hook directly onto the archwire.
    - ○ Removable appliances: loops on an upper removable appliance (URA) allow attachment of headgear.
- Neck strap or headcap (extra-oral fitting):
  - Neck strap: this is used for cervical (low) pull and combi (straight) pull headgear (Figure 29.5).
  - Headcap: this is used for high pull headgear.
- Elastic component or spring mechanism
  - This connects the other two elements and controls the magnitude of the force applied.

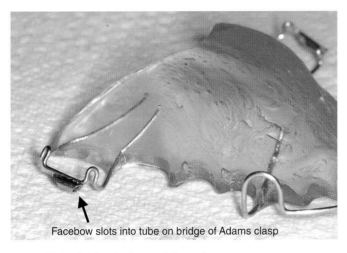

Facebow slots into tube on bridge of Adams clasp

Figure 29.4 Soldered tubes on Adams clasp.

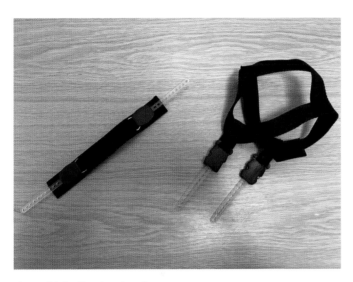

Figure 29.5 Head and neck strap.

– Elastic force is produced by:
  ○ Elastic strap
  ○ Different sizes of extra-oral elastic bands
  ○ Spring mechanisms.

29.7 Headgear Injuries and Preventative Measures

Injuries can occur with the use of headgear, especially to the soft tissues such as eyes, eyelids, nose, and lips. In 1994, nine serious injuries from headgear were recorded; after these incidents headgear had to have at least two safety features (one extra-oral, one intra-oral), which helped prevent further injuries occurring. The most common injury is ocular injury and the most severe injury is total blindness.

Injury can occur when a facebow is used with elastics for the mechanism. If the facebow is pulled out of the intra-oral attachment, the springback mechanism can make the facebow recoil into the facial soft tissues.

The British Orthodontic Society (BOS) recommends that all headgear used must have at least two or more safety mechanisms:

- One extra-oral
- One intra-oral.

The different types of safety mechanisms are:

- Recurved safety facebow (intra-oral): facebow with blunt ends which may reduce the incidence of any penetrating injuries.
- Rigid masal strap (extra-oral): this helps prevent the facebow from being dislodged (Figure 29.6).
- Snap-away modules (spring mechanism, extra-oral): built into the headgear strap where it attaches to the facebow (Figure 29.7). If excessive force is applied the components come apart, preventing recoil of the facebow.
- Locking facebow (intra-oral; Figure 29.8):
  - Prevents any trauma from sharp ends.
  - In addition a facebow has been developed with a small catch to lock it into the molar tubes, which prevents it from being pulled out.

If headgear is used without any safety mechanism it is considered negligence towards the patient.

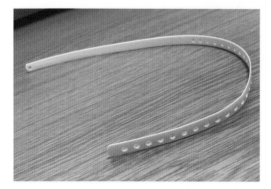

Figure 29.6 Masal strap.

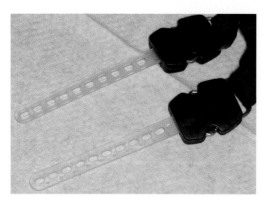

Figure 29.7 Snap-away modules.

Figure 29.8   Locking intra-oral facebow.

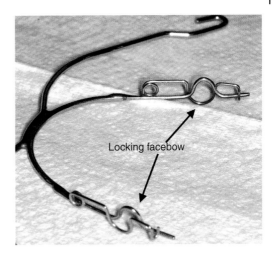

Locking facebow

All patients should be warned of the dangers of headgear and instructed that it should not be worn during contact sports. If headgear dislodges during the night, patients should be informed to stop wear and return it for adjustment by the clinician.

One disadvantage of wearing headgear with a removable appliance is that the Adams clasp can become distorted, causing the headgear to dislodge. If this happens the patient must return to the orthodontist as soon as possible to have it looked at.

29.8   Reverse Headgear

Reverse headgear is also known as a facemask and is used on class III cases, such as:

- Where forward movement of the maxilla is needed.
- To move teeth mesially to close up any excess spacing.

This type of headgear stops the mandible from protruding forward and the forehead is used as the resistance.

29.9   Assessment of Wear

At appointments it is important to assess whether your patient has been wearing their headgear. However, sometimes it can be difficult to tell if they have done as instructed. These points can help determine whether they have done as instructed:

- They bring it to every appointment.
- They can fit it easily themselves.
- You can see the neck or head strap has been used.
- Teeth are moving/mobile.
- They keep asking for more elastics.
- They can do a chart for number of hours of wear.
- A new size of facebow is required due to the teeth moving.

29.10 Measuring Force

Force is measured by the use of a correx gauge. There are two different sizes of correx gauges, big and smaller (Figures 29.9 and 29.10). The big gauge is used for measuring forces on headgear, and the small gauge is used for measuring the forces of extra-oral or intra-oral elastics.

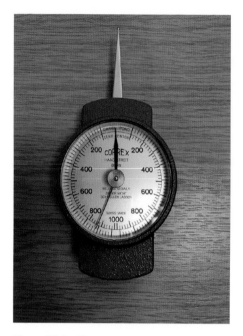

Figure 29.9 Big correx gauge.

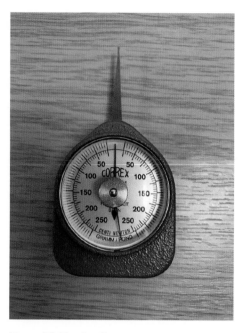

Figure 29.10 Small correx gauge.

30

Instructions for all Appliances

30.1 Removable Appliances

- The appliance must be worn full time, including at night.
- The appliance can be worn when eating, but it should be removed after to clean before inserting back into the mouth.
- The appliance must be removed for contact sports and for playing a musical instrument, etc.
- The appliance must be removed and cleaned twice a day when cleaning teeth (morning and night) with the use of a toothbrush and toothpaste or Retainer Brite.
- Show the patient how to insert and remove the appliance.
- Show the patient how to adjust the appliance if needed, for example with a midline expansion screw, insert the key and turn once a week (one quarter turn once a week, resulting in 0.25 mm).
- The appliance must be brought to every appointment and be well looked after – if the appliance is broken and needs replacing, this can incur a cost.
- Teeth may be tender for anything up to a week when they are starting to move and the appliance may rub on the inside of the cheek. This occurs as the mouth is getting used to having the appliance – use warm salty water for any ulcers, Bonjela only over the age of 16 years, and paracetamol, Calpol, Nurofen, etc. for any pain.
- If there are any problems the patient must call the practice.

30.2 Functional Appliances

- The appliance must be worn full time, including at night.
- The appliance is to be worn when eating, but removed after to clean, before inserting back into the mouth. This allows for the appliance to work more efficiently.
- The appliance must be removed for contact sports, musical instruments, etc.
- The appliance must be removed and cleaned twice a day when cleaning teeth (morning and night), with the use of a toothbrush and toothpaste or Retainer Brite.
- Show the patient how to insert and remove the appliance.
- Show the patient how to adjust the appliance if needed, for example for a modified twin block with a midline expansion screw, insert the key and turn once a week (one quarter turn once a week resulting in 0.25 mm).

Textbook for Orthodontic Therapists, First Edition. Ceri Davies.
© 2020 John Wiley & Sons Ltd. Published 2020 by John Wiley & Sons Ltd.

- The appliance must be brought to every appointment and well looked after – if it is broken and needs replacing, this can incur a cost.
- Teeth and jaws may start to ache by the evening after fitting the appliance and can last up to about a week. Reassure the patient that this is normal, as it is just where the appliance is starting to work. Pain relief tablets such as paracetamol, Nurofen, Calpol, etc. can be taken.
- If there are any problems the patient must call the practice.

30.3 Fixed Appliances

- Reassure the patient that although the appliance will feel strange, they will get used to it in a couple of days.
- The teeth may feel tender by the evening after fitting the appliance. This is perfectly normal, as it is just where the teeth are starting to move. This can last anything up to a week, so paracetamol, Nurofen, ibuprofen, etc, will help.
- The appliance may also start to rub the inside of the cheek and ulcers may appear. This is also normal, as it is just where the mouth is getting used to having the brace. This can last anything up to about a week and will settle down. Advise that rinsing with warm salty water in the tender area will help to settle down any ulcers or that Bonjela can be used if the patient is over 16 years. Ibuprofen will also help to settle down any inflammation. Orthodontic wax is helpful to use by placing it over the area of the brace that is rubbing; it will ease the gum on the inside and stop the brace from irritating the cheek.
- Avoid any bright or richly coloured foods for 24 hours after a fixed brace is fitted, as they may stain the teeth permanently, for example ketchup, soup, brown sauce, mustard, baked beans, curries, etc. The patient can have water, milk, lemonade, plain pasta, white cheese, potatoes, fish, chips, and any bland-coloured foods.

30.4 Cleaning Instructions for the Patient

- *Orthodontic brush/conventional brush*:
  - Spend four minutes every morning and evening cleaning your teeth and brace.
  - Spend two minutes on your teeth, doing circular motions on each tooth for three seconds.
  - Spend two minutes on your brace, ensuring you are cleaning under the archwires and around the brackets and bands.
- *Interspace brush*
  - Use this brush to clean underneath each archwire between the brackets to remove any plaque or food debris.
- *Tepee brushes*
  - Use these brushes to clean around each side of the bracket. This will remove any plaque build-up and food debris. It will also prevent staining around the brackets, which can lead to decalcification.
  - If an appropriate size is chosen these brushes can also be used between the teeth as an alternative to floss.
- *Floss*
  - Floss can be used to clean around the brackets as an alternative to the tepee brushes.
  - Floss can also be used by feeding it underneath the archwire and between the teeth to clean the contact points and gum margin.

- *Mouthwash*
  - Fluoride mouthwash should not be used for the first three days as it could permanently stain your teeth. After that mouthwash should be used twice a day, ideally late morning and late afternoon for a fluoride intake throughout the day.
- *Disclosing tablets*
  - Disclosing tablets should not be used for the first three days as it could permanently stain your teeth. These tablets should occasionally be used to make sure you are cleaning properly. Chew on the tablet for about a minute after cleaning and then spit it out. Any areas of dark purple and light purple are built-up areas of plaque that have been missed when cleaning.
- *Diet*
  - Foods to avoid that cause breakages include:
    - Hard/sticky foods and fizzy drinks.
    - For example crusty bread, toffees, hard nuts, bubblegum/chewing gum, pizza crusts.
- *Orthodontic wax*
  - Wax can be used on the area of the brace that is rubbing the cheek. If a long wire causes irritation, either cut it yourself using nail clippers or place wax on the end of the archwire. Loose brackets that may cause irritation can also have wax placed on them to prevent them from swinging around on the archwire. By pulling off a bit of wax and rolling it into a ball, it can be pushed and placed around the archwire and left there. It will not cause any harm if swallowed.
- *Call the practice*
  - If there are any problems such as the following you must call the practice:
    - Loose bracket
    - Long wire
    - Irritation to the gums
    - Loose ligature/module
    - Loose hook for elastic wear.

30.5 Headgear

- Show the patient how to place and remove the appliance in the mirror.
- Advise the patient to bring it to every appointment.
- The appliance has to be worn every single night for 10–12 hours for anchorage or 14–16 hours for traction.
- Explain the risks of injuries and how they can happen.
- Headgear should be removed for sports.
- Remove the appliance when cleaning teeth and clean it with toothbrush and toothpaste.
- If headgear dislodges at night, then call the practice *as soon as possible* to stop any further injuries that could occur from – they should cease treatment straight away until they have seen the orthodontist.

30.6 Retainers

- The retainer has to be worn every single night for 10–12 hours. If the patient is not sleeping for that long, extra time must be made up in the evening after dinner.
- The retainer is cleaned every single morning with the use of a non-abrasive toothpaste and toothbrush or with Retainer Brite.

- Explain to the patient that if the retainer is not worn every single night, the teeth will move back to how they were before treatment. As the NHS only pays for one course of treatment, any re-treatment will have to be paid for privately.
- The retainer is to be kept in its box when not being worn and kept out of the way of pets, especially dogs, as they love the smell of saliva!
- The NHS only supplies retainers once, so if they have been lost or the dog has eaten them, a new set will need to be paid for.
- The retainer must be brought to every retention check appointment to see how it is fitting.
- If there are any problems then the patient must call the practice.

30.7   Bonded Retainers

- Bonded retainers are fixed to the teeth and cannot be removed by the patient.
- A bonded retainer must be kept clean when cleaning the teeth. The teeth should be cleaned as normal behind the teeth where the bonded retainer is. Floss or Tepee brushes should be used and threaded through the contact points of the teeth, so that any food or plaque that has got caught around the bonded retainer can be removed.
- Removable retainers must still be worn every single night for 10–12 hours: the teeth are liable to move as the bonded retainer is only holding the front six teeth.
- If the bonded retainer comes loose, the patient must call the practice straight away and must wear the removable retainer full time until they come in and have it repaired. If it is lost a charge will be made for its replacement.
- Biting into hard foods can cause the bonded retainer to dislodge and become loose, so the patient should avoid biting into hard foods such as apples, crusty rolls, etc.
- If there are any problems the patient must contact the practice.

31

Uncommon Removable Appliances

31.1 Nudger Appliance

The nudger appliance is a type of upper removable appliance (URA) that is used in orthodontics. This appliance is used in conjunction with headgear that is attached to molar bands and consists of:

- Adams clasps on the upper first premolars.
- Palatal finger springs mesial to the upper first permanent molars.
- A Southend clasp around the upper central incisors.
- A flat anterior bite plane (FABP), which will help to decrease an increased overbite by disarticulating the posterior teeth.

This appliance is considered when bilateral molar movement is required, as the palatal finger springs that lay mesial to the upper first permanent molar will help to distalise them with the use of headgear. Patients presenting with deepbites will also benefit from this appliance as it incorporates an FABP. This helps to decrease a deepbite/increased overbite. The nudger appliance should not be considered without the use of headgear, because it can result in loss of anchorage. However, the nudger appliance must be worn full time, even though headgear will only be worn for 12–14 hours. When taking an impression for the appliance, the molar bands must first be cemented in situ.

The nudger appliance consists of active and retentive components, anchorage, and baseplate:

- *Active*: to achieve distalisation of the upper first molars, palatal finger springs lie mesially to UR6 and UL6. These springs will help to distalise the upper first molars and place a force on these teeth alongside the use of headgear.
- *Retention*: two types of retentive components are considered, Adam's clasps on the upper first premolars and Southend clasps on the upper central incisors. These components are used to help retain the appliance in the mouth.
- *Anchorage*: Every action has an equal and opposite reaction, therefore anchorage in this case is very important. Anchorage can be found from the baseplate. Palatal finger springs are used to help distalise the upper first molars, but this can have an effect on the rest of the dentition, as mesial movement can occur resulting in an increased overjet. Headgear provides the main force for distalising the upper first permanent molars, but it is only worn at night, so when it is not worn the appliance acts as a retainer, with the palatal finger springs maintaining the movement that has been achieved with headgear.

Textbook for Orthodontic Therapists, First Edition. Ceri Davies.

- *Baseplate*: the acrylic baseplate helps to house and support the active and retentive components on the appliance. As well as distalising the upper first molars, it also helps to correct deepbites, therefore an FABP is needed. This achieves 2 mm of disarticulation of the posterior segment, allowing these teeth to extrude to help open the bite anteriorly. Collets of acrylic are found around the teeth on the baseplate of a removable appliance. This should be removed from the distal aspect of the molars and second premolars, which will allow for distalisation of these teeth. Without it being removed, movement cannot be achieved.

31.2 En Masse Appliance

This type of appliance is only worn at night and has headgear directly incorporated into it. The appliance is to encourage closure of an anterior open bite with the use of headgear. The design consists of Adams clasps on the upper first molars and premolars, a midline coffin spring, and a facebow for headgear joining onto the tubes of the Adams clasps on the first premolar.

31.3 ACCO Appliance

ACCO stands for acrylic-cervical-occipital. Headgear is incorporated with the appliance, which helps to achieve distalisation of the molars and to reduce a deepbite. Cervical low pull headgear would be considered with this appliance, as it will extrude the upper molars to open the deepbite.
  Design of the ACCO appliance:

- Adams clasps on the first premolars to aid retention.
- Southend clasp on the upper central incisors to aid retention.
- Palatal springs mesial to banded first permanent molars – active component.
- FABP to open the deepbite.

31.4 ELSAA

ELSAA stands for expansion, labial segment aligning appliance. This is used prior to functional appliance treatment and especially for class II div II cases. This type of appliance can be another alternative at the start of treatment in such cases. Instead of either using a sectional fixed or URA with an active component to procline the upper central incisors, the ELSAA will help to procline the upper incisors, expand the posterior dentition, and reduce the overbite.
  Design of the ELSAA:

- Adams clasps on the first permanent molars and first premolars – retentive component.
- Midline expansion screw – active component to expand upper posterior dentition.
- FABP to help reduce a deepbite.
- Double cantilever spring (Z spring) behind upper central incisors – active component to procline upper central incisors.

32

Anchorage

Anchorage is the control of unwanted tooth movement. Anchorage works by Newton's Third Law – to every action there is an equal and opposite reaction.

Anchorage is needed throughout orthodontic treatment, including for:

- Alignment
- Levelling
- Overjet and overbite correction
- Space closure
- Retention

There are two types of anchorage:

- Intra-oral
- Extra-oral.

32.1 Intra-oral Anchorage

32.1.1 Simple Anchorage

This type of anchorage is where there is active movement of one tooth pulled against several anchor teeth. For example, Figure 32.1 shows that lower second permanent molars have been extracted and space closure is needed. When undertying L6-6, this acts as an anchor unit and stops movement of the lower first permanent molars, allowing space closure of the second permanent molars.

32.1.2 Compound Anchorage

The resistance provided by more than one tooth with greater support is used to move teeth with less support. Teeth with a smaller root surface area are pitted against teeth with a larger root surface area. There is more than one tooth within the anchor unit.

For example, in Figure 32.2, upper canines were favoured for extraction and space closure was needed. By undertying U7s–U4s, both sides will act as an anchor unit, preventing mesial movement of these teeth and allowing the retraction of the anterior segment. Another example would be if upper first premolars were extracted, undertying U7s–U5s on both sides with chain elastic U5-5 would help retract the anterior segment.

Textbook for Orthodontic Therapists, First Edition. Ceri Davies.
© 2020 John Wiley & Sons Ltd. Published 2020 by John Wiley & Sons Ltd.

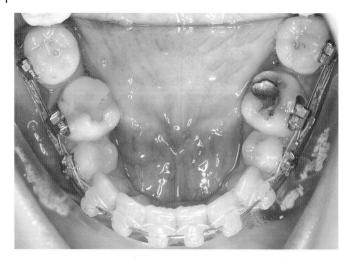

Figure 32.1 Lower occlusal showing simple anchorage. Undertie on L6-6 (anchor unit) with L8s being brought forward via chain elastic against several anchor teeth.

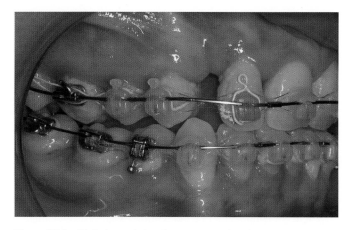

Figure 32.2 Right buccal showing compound anchorage.

32.1.3 Stationary Anchorage

This type of anchorage is the strongest, however it is rarely used nowadays as not many orthodontists use temporary anchorage devices (TADs) and ankylosed teeth are seldom seen. With stationary anchorage it is difficult to prevent movement of the anchor teeth all together, as you can never get 100% anchorage. Tipping versus bodily movement of teeth can be seen with this type of anchorage, for instance with retraction of incisors when using the molar teeth as an anchor unit with class II elastics.

Figure 32.3 shows two types of stationary anchorage with the use of TADs and ankylosed teeth.

32.1.4 Reciprocal Anchorage

This type of anchorage is when two teeth, or two groups of teeth, move in equal and opposite directions. Examples would be an upper removable appliance (URA) with midline expansion screw, quadhelix, rapid maxillary expansion (RME), crossbite elastics on both sides, transpalatal arch (TPA), TPA with Nance, and lingual arch. Figure 32.4 illustrates various types of mechanics.

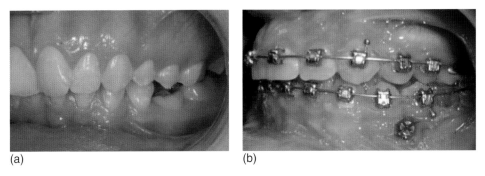

Figure 32.3 Temporary anchorage devices (TADs) and ankylosed lower left deciduous molar showing stationary anchorage. (a) Ankylosis: tooth is fused to the bone and cannot move due to no periodontal ligament. Does not respond to orthodontic forces. (b) TAD is placed into the bone and cannot move.

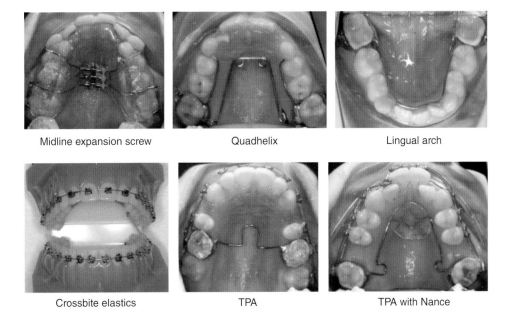

| Midline expansion screw | Quadhelix | Lingual arch |

| Crossbite elastics | TPA | TPA with Nance |

Figure 32.4 Different types of reciprocal anchorage. TPA, transpalatal arch.

32.2 Extra-Oral Anchorage

Extra-oral anchorage can also be considered and the patient wearing headgear achieves this. It will apply a distal force on the molars and the patient's head is used for anchorage.

32.3 What Does Anchorage Depend On?

Anchorage can depend on different factors such as:

- The number of teeth that need to be moved:
  - The more teeth that need to be moved, the greater the demand on anchorage.

- The distance the teeth need to be moved:
  - This depends on how far the teeth need to be moved and whether it is anterior or posterior movement.
  - The bigger the distance, the greater the demand on anchorage.
- Aims of treatment:
  - The aims of treatment depend on how severe the case is.
  - The more severe the case, the more anchorage is required.
  - The less severe the case, the less anchorage is required.
- Type of tooth movement planned:
  - Bodily movement and tipping movement require different levels of anchorage.
  - Bodily movement produces more force, meaning more anchorage is needed, for example for space closure.
  - Tipping movement produces less force, meaning less anchorage is needed, for example class II elastics retracting upper anterior segment in round archwires.
- Root surface area of teeth used for anchorage:
  - Teeth all have different root surface areas, for example single-rooted teeth have less root surface area than multirooted teeth.
  - Therefore, teeth with a greater root surface area are harder to move, but easier to keep in place. They will produce a better anchor unit, as if these teeth need to move they will apply a greater force on anchorage.
- Skeletal pattern:
  - The skeletal pattern can have an effect on anchorage loss.
  - Patients presenting with an increased vertical skeletal pattern and a backward growth rotation have the risk of experiencing more anchorage loss than patients with a decreased vertical skeletal pattern and a forward growth rotation. This is because each different facial type has different muscular strength, one having good strength and the other not.
- Occlusal interlock:
  - Good intercuspation at the end of treatment can help prevent anchorage loss.
  - It is important to ensure that all teeth have good interdigitation; however, this may be difficult to achieve in some cases depending on whether a tooth/teeth need(s) to be moved.
- Tendency for tooth movement in the arch:
  - Anchorage loss can occur more in the upper arch as there is more risk of mesial drift.

32.4   Reinforcing Anchorage

Increasing anchorage can be achieved in the following ways:

- Increasing the number of teeth in the anchor unit:
  - Increasing the anchor unit by adding more teeth to it can help to prevent unwanted movement of active teeth.
  - More teeth being included in the anchor unit results in more force.
- Making movement of anchor teeth more difficult:
  - Bodily movement versus tipping movement.
  - It is important to think of what movement is required when needing to reinforce anchorage.
  - Tipping movement results in less chance of anchorage loss.
  - Bodily movement results in more chance of anchorage loss.

- Intermaxillary elastics:
  - Intermaxillary elastics such as class II and class III use the opposing arch to reinforce anchorage.
  - Elastics will act as an anchor unit to help pull teeth anteriorly/posteriorly depending on the class of elastics, for example:
    - Class II intermaxillary elastics – undertie upper 3-3 to prevent gaps appearing and hold teeth in position.
    - Class III intermaxillary elastics – undertie lower 3-3 to prevent gaps appearing and hold teeth in position.
- Palatal and lingual arches:
  - TPA (Figure 32.5):
    - Constructed in 0.9 mm stainless-steel wire that transverses the hard palate and is attached to molar bands that are cemented to the first molars.
    - Stops the upper first and second permanent molars from moving mesially as soon as the mesio-buccal root of the upper first permanent molars hits cortical bone.
    - The arch is connected to molar bands which fix the maxillary intermolar width and help prevent these teeth from moving mesially.
  - TPA with Nance (Figure 32.6):
    - Constructed in 0.9 mm stainless-steel wire.
    - Extends to the palatal vault via molar bands and incorporates an acrylic button that lies on the palatal mucosa.
    - Helps fix the upper arch length and stops the upper first and second permanent molars moving mesially through resistance from either maxillary vault or basal bone (mainly the former), acting as a barrier.
    - Pressure is placed on the Nance button to stop mesial movement of the upper first and second permanent molars.
    - Acrylic Nance is immovable and does not change.
    - A common problem is that gingiva can form over the acrylic when applying too much force, which results in the Nance being embedded in the palate.

Figure 32.5 Transpalatal arch.

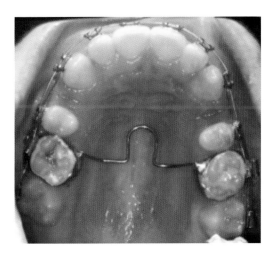

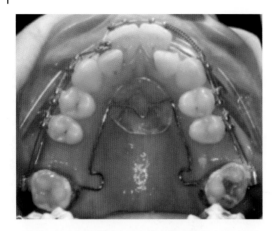

Figure 32.6 Transpalatal arch with Nance button.

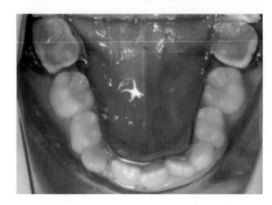

Figure 32.7 Lingual arch.

- – Lingual arch (Figure 32.7):
  - o Constructed in 0.9 mm stainless-steel wire.
  - o Used in the mandibular arch.
  - o The wire extends behind the lower incisors of the lingual surface of the teeth and extends to the molar bands cemented on the first molars.
  - o Resistance comes from the lower incisors.
  - o Stops 6s and 7s moving mesially.
  - o Generally used as a space maintainer.
- • Choice of appliance:
  - – Different appliances can offer more anchorage than others. For example, due to the palatal coverage of a removable appliance, it will provide more anchorage than a fixed appliance.
  - – Implants:
  - – Implants provide a good source of anchorage because they are stuck in the bone and cannot move.
  - – This type of anchorage is good for patients with hypodontia or ankylosis.
  - – Other types of implants that can be used for orthodontic treatment re:
    - o Micro-implants
    - o Palatal implants
    - o Mini-plates
    - o Mini-screws – TADs

32.5   Sources of Anchorage

Consideration of the following can help with anchorage:

- Bonding 7s
- TPA/TPA with Nance
- TADs – stationary anchorage
- Implants
- Extra-oral anchorage (headgear)
- URA baseplate
- Intermaxillary elastics
- Stopped arches – V notch in archwire prevents teeth moving forward
- Ankylosed teeth
- Lingual arches
- Root surface area
- Mucosa or bone.

32.6   Anchorage Loss

Anchorage loss is where undesirable tooth movement happens and this can be seen in all three planes of space:

- Antero-posterior – front to back
- Vertical – up and down
- Transverse - side to side.

An example of anchorage loss is where posterior teeth move forward instead of incisors moving back when reducing an overjet. However, there are many other reasons why there could be anchorage loss, such as:

- Forces that are too heavy
- Maxillary arch more susceptible
- Occlusal interferences
- Vertical growth pattern
- Poor patient compliance:
  - Patients with a URA can suffer anchorage loss if it is not worn full time.
  - Poor compliance can result in forward movement of molars leading to loss of anchorage.
  - Fixed appliances with breakages, failure to wear headgear, and elastic traction all lead to anchorage loss.
  - Anchorage is easy to lose, so monitor patient compliance on every visit.

33

Index of Orthodontic Treatment Need (IOTN)

The IOTN is the Index of Orthodontic Treatment Need and has two components:

- Dental Health Component (DHC)
- Aesthetic Component (AC).

It assesses the *worst* feature of the malocclusion and the need for treatment. It is used as a government initiative to assess patients' need for orthodontic treatment on the NHS.

The IOTN can be used by NHS practices and clinicians who are suitably qualified, and can be used in clinical assessment, at chairside, and on study models.

33.1   Dental Health Component

This component looks at the worst feature of the malocclusion that has an impact on dental health. It operates by the following the acronym that helps to identify the worst occlusal feature, MOCDO:

M – Missing
O – Overjet/reverse overjet
C – Crossbites
D – Displacement in contact points
O – Overbite/openbites

Once the worst feature has been identified, it is then initialised with a letter, as follows:

a – Overjet
i – Impeded or impacted teeth
m & b – Reverse overjet
p – Cleft lip and palate
s – Submerged deciduous teeth

h – Hypodontia
l – Lingual crossbite
t – Tipped teeth
x – Supernumerary
g – Good occlusion
c – Crossbites
d – Displacement of contact points

Textbook for Orthodontic Therapists, First Edition. Ceri Davies.
© 2020 John Wiley & Sons Ltd. Published 2020 by John Wiley & Sons Ltd.

e – Openbites/anterior openbites (AOB)
f – Overbites/deepbites

After initialisation there are five grades within the DHC into which the patient can be classified. The grading all depends on if their worst feature meets the requirements of that grade:

Grade 5 – Very great need
Grade 4 – Great need
Grade 3 – Borderline need (AC component used)
Grade 2 – Little need
Grade 1 – No need

Regardless of MOCDO, the highest grade is always chosen. For instance, if there is one occlusal anomaly in grade 5 and the rest in grade 4, it would be grade 5.

33.1.1 Grade 5

5i – Impeded or impacted teeth
5h – More than one missing tooth in any quadrant
5a – Overjet >9 mm
5m – Reverse overjet >3.5 mm with masticatory/speech difficulties
5p – Cleft lip and palate
5s – Submerged deciduous teeth

33.1.2 Grade 4

4h – Only one missing tooth in any quadrant
4b – Reverse overjet >3.5 mm with no masticatory/speech difficulties
4m – Reverse overjet >1 mm but <3.5 mm with masticatory/speech difficulties
4c – Anterior and posterior crossbites with >2 mm displacement between retruded contact position (RCP) and intercuspal position (ICP)
4L – Posterior lingual crossbite
4d – Contact point displacement >4 mm
4e – Extreme lateral openbites or AOB >4 mm
4f – Increased and complete overbite with trauma
4t – Tipped teeth, partially erupted
4a – Overjet >6 mm or = 9 mm
4x – Supernumerary present

33.1.3 Grade 3

3a – Overjet >3.5 mm with incompetent lips
3b – Reverse overjet >1 mm
3c – Anterior and posterior crossbites >1 mm between RCP and ICP
3d – Contact point displacement >2 mm
3e – Lateral openbite or AOB >2 mm
3f – Deepbite and complete to gingival or palatal tissues with no trauma

33.1.4 Grade 2

2a – Overjet >3.5 mm with competent lips
2b – Reverse overjet >0 mm but ≤1 mm
2c – Anterior and posterior crossbites ≤1 mm between RCP and ICP
2d – Contact point displacement ≥1 mm or <2 mm
2e – AOB and posterior openbite (POB) >1 mm but ≤2 mm
2f – Increased overbite ≥3.5 mm with no gingival contact
2g – Pre- or post-normal occlusion with no other anomalies – good occlusion

33.1.5 Grade 1

Minor malocclusions including contact point displacement <1 mm

33.1.6 RCP and ICP

RCP and ICP look at how the teeth meet on occluding:

- **Retruded contact position** (also known as centric relation): the position at which the teeth meet first before deviating into complete intercuspation.
- **Intercuspal position** (also known as centric occlusion): complete intercuspation of the opposing teeth.

The molars meet cusp to cusp on closing (RCP), then deviate into complete intercuspation (ICP).

33.2 Aesthetic Component

This component is used in conjunction with grade 3 and assesses the impact of the appearance of the malocclusion to the patient. This determines the patient's level of psychological damage.

If a patient qualifies for a grade 3, a set of 10 colour photographs of different levels of attractiveness of malocclusions is used (Figure 33.1). The clinician then assesses the patient's malocclusion by picking a photograph that they think best represents their malocclusion. Depending on which they pick:

- Photograph 1–5 *do not* qualify for treatment.
- Photograph 6–10 *do* qualify for treatment.

The disadvantage of the photographs is that they are all the same, just presenting more crowding. There are no examples of AOB, class III malocclusion, POB, and so on.

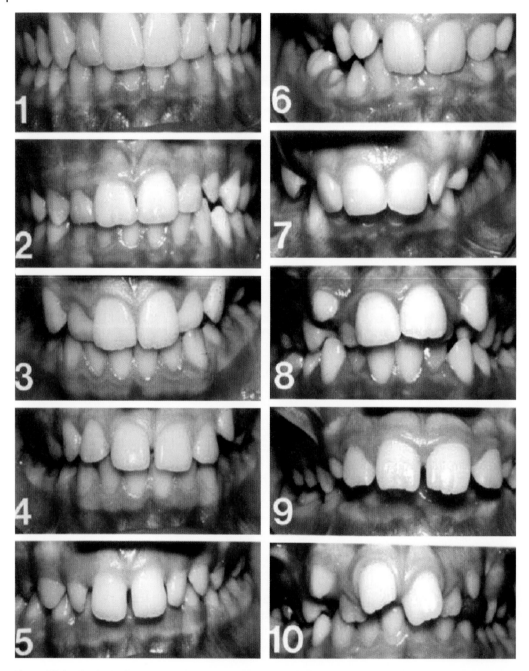

Figure 33.1 Aesthetic Component of the Index of Orthodontic Treatment Need: The SCAN scale. *Source:* Ruth Evans and William Shaw (1987). Preliminary evaluation of an illustrated scale for rating dental attractiveness. *European Journal of Orthodontics* 9(4): 314–318. Reproduced by permission of Oxford University Press.

34

Peer Assessment Rating (PAR)

The Peer Assessment Rating or (PAR) is used to measure the success of treatment. It is used on pre-treatment and post-treatment study models, for the following reasons:

- To measure the success and lack of success of treatment.
- To help improve the quality of treatment.
- As a cumulative score: the difference between the pre- and post-treatment PAR scores indicates the degree of improvement as a result of orthodontic treatment. Figure 34.1 shows the scoring sheet.

34.1 Components of PAR

There are five components of PAR:

1) Upper and lower anterior segments
2) Right and left buccal segments
3) Overjet and reversed overjet
4) Overbite and openbite
5) Centreline.

All the PAR components in each section are scored, added up and given an unweighted total. The unweighted total in each section is then multiplied by the relevant weighting factor (Table 34.1) to give an overall weighted total for each section:

Total for component × Weighting factor = Weighted total

The weighted totals for all components need to be added together to give the total PAR score for both pre- and post-study models.

34.1.1 Upper and Lower Anterior Segments

- Looks at contact point displacement upper and lower 3-3.
- Each study model is measured and held looking from the occlusal plane.
- A PAR ruler (Figure 34.2) is used on the contact point section.

Textbook for Orthodontic Therapists, First Edition. Ceri Davies.
© 2020 John Wiley & Sons Ltd. Published 2020 by John Wiley & Sons Ltd.

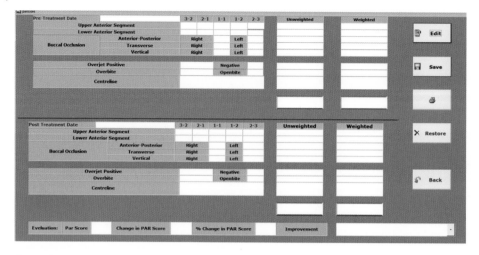

Figure 34.1 Example of a PAR scoring sheet on DOIT software.

Table 34.1 Weighting factors of each component.

Component 1: Upper and lower anterior segments	×1
Component 2: Right and left buccal segments	×1
Component 3: Overjet	×6
Component 4: Overbite	×2
Component 5: Centreline	×4

- The lines on this section are positioned to lie across the teeth in the antero-posterior (AP) plane. This line is scored by measuring the line of best fit between the contact points on the mesial and distal aspects of where they should meet.
- They score between 1 and 5.
- The scores are added up and multiplied by their weighting factor ×1.

34.1.2 Right and Left Buccal Segments

- Looks at the buccal occlusion on the right and left sides on teeth 3–7 in all three planes – AP, vertical and transverse.
- The study model is put in its correct occlusion:
  - AP plane:
    - Teeth (3–7) both sides
    - Looks at the molar relationship
    - Scored as:
      - 0 = Good interdigitation (full unit class I, II, III)

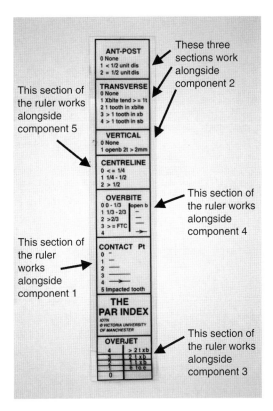

This section of the ruler works alongside component 5

ANT-POST
0 None
1 < 1/2 unit dis
2 = 1/2 unit dis

These three sections work alongside component 2

TRANSVERSE
0 None
1 Xbite tend > = 1t
2 1 tooth in xbite
3 > 1 tooth in xb
4 > 1 tooth in sb

VERTICAL
0 None
1 openb 2t > 2mm

CENTRELINE
0 < = 1/4
1 1/4 - 1/2
2 > 1/2

OVERBITE
0 0 - 1/3   open b
1 1/3 - 2/3   —
2 > 2/3   —
3 > = FTC   —
4   →

This section of the ruler works alongside component 4

CONTACT Pt
0 —
1 —
2 —
3 —
4 →
5 Impacted tooth

This section of the ruler works alongside component 1

THE
PAR INDEX
IOTN
© VICTORIA UNIVERSITY
OF MANCHESTER

OVERJET
4   > 2 1 xb
3   2 1 xb
2   1 1 xb
1   e to e
0

This section of the ruler works alongside component 3

Figure 34.2 PAR ruler.

- 1 = <½ unit from full interdigitation (II1/4, II3/4, III1/4, III3/4)
- 2 = ½ unit cusp to cusp (II1/2, III1/2)
 – Vertical plane:
   ○ Teeth (3–7) both sides
   ○ Looks for any posterior openbite (POB)
   ○ Scored as:
     • 0 = None
     • 1 = Lateral openbite on 2 or more teeth >2 mm
 – Transverse plane:
   ○ Teeth (3–7) both sides
   ○ Looks for any crossbites
   ○ Scored as:
     • 0 = None
     • 1 = Crossbite tendency
     • 2 = 1 tooth in crossbite
     • 3 = >1 tooth in crossbite
     • 4 = >1 tooth in scissorbite
 • Each plane is scored and added up separately and multiplied by the weighting factor of ×1.

34.1.3 Overjet and Reversed Overjet

- Looks at anterior segment in occlusion.
- Measures positive and negative overjet:
  - Positive overjet:
    - ○ Measured from the most prominent incisor.
    - ○ PAR ruler held parallel to the occlusal plane using the overjet section.
    - ○ See which box the most prominent incisor sits in, if it sits on a line take the lower score.
    - ○ Scored as 0, 1, 2, 3, or 4.
  - Negative overjet:
    - ○ Looks for any anterior crossbites.
    - ○ Negative overjet scored as:
      - 0 = No crossbite
      - 1 = 1 or >1 tooth edge to edge
      - 2 = 1 tooth in crossbite
      - 3 = 2 teeth in crossbite
      - 4 = >2 teeth in crossbite
- Each occlusal feature is scored and added up separately and multiplied by the weighting factor of ×6.

34.1.4 Overbite and Openbite

- Looks at the anterior segment in occlusion.
  - Overbite:
    - ○ Recorded vertically on the greatest coverage of the lower incisors.
    - ○ Scores are made up in thirds.
    - ○ Lower incisor visually divided up into horizontal thirds.
    - ○ Score assessed by how many thirds the upper incisors cover.
    - ○ Scores calculated as:
      - 0 = <1/3 coverage
      - 1 = >1/3 and <2/3 coverage
      - 2 = >2/3 coverage
      - 3 = Full tooth coverage
  - Openbite:
    - ○ Recorded between incisal edges.
    - ○ Openbite section used on PAR ruler.
    - ○ Lines placed vertically between upper and lower incisor edges.
    - ○ Line of best fit given a score:
      - 0 = No anterior openbite (AOB)
      - 1 = ≤1 mm
      - 2 = 1.1–2 mm
      - 3 = 2.1–4 mm
      - 4 = >4.1 mm
- Each occlusal feature is scored and added up separately and then multiplied by the weighting factor of ×2.

34.1.5 Centreline

- Looks at the relation of the upper centreline in relation to the lower centreline.
- Looks at the anterior segment in occlusion.
- Scores made up into quarters.
- Lower incisor divided into vertical quarters.
- Upper centreline then worked out by how many quarters it is off relative to the lower incisor.
- Scores calculated as:
  - 0 = <1/4
  - 1 = 1/4–1/2
  - 2 = >1/2
- Scores added up and multiplied by the weighting factor of ×4.

34.2 Assessment of Improvement in PAR

Since PAR is used to measure the success of treatment, calculations are carried out on each patient's initial and final study models to work out the overall percentage of improvement. The calculations for this are as follows:

- Record the *starting PAR*
- Record the *finishing PAR*
- Work out the *reduction in PAR:*

  Starting PAR – Finishing PAR

- % Reduction:

  $$\left(\text{Reduction} \div \text{starting PAR}\right) \times 100 = \text{percentage reduction}$$

  70% is a good standard

- Less than 5 PAR points for final study model = excellent occlusion.
- More than 10 PAR points for final study model = unacceptable occlusion.
- Remember:
  - Scores are cumulative, unlike in the IOTN.
  - 10 or fewer PAR points = greatly improved.
- If you lose the pre-study model for a particular patient, a finishing PAR score of 10 or less signifies a great improvement.

34.3 Who Uses PAR?

Any member of the orthodontic team can PAR score, especially team members who have undergone special training in how to achieve the ratings. PAR is used on pre- and post-treatment study models for all patients who have undergone orthodontic treatment on the NHS. Primary Care Trusts use this method to assess treatment outcomes each year on a sample of more than 30 cases.

Orthodontists are allowed to have 5% of cases graded as no improvement, but if more than 5% of all their cases are deemed to be graded as no improvement, then this is a very poor result.

35

Space Analysis

Space analysis is used in orthodontics to work out the amount of space that is required in each dental arch. This process is used prior to starting treatment to ensure that the treatment aims are appropriate to the patient.

Space is required to correct the following:

- Crowding.
- Incisor antero-posterior (AP) change (to achieve a normal overjet of 2 mm).
- Levelling of occlusal curves.
- Arch expansion (to create space).
- Correction of upper incisor angulation (mesiodistal tip).
- Correction of upper incisor inclination (torque).

35.1 Crowding

The amount of crowding present can be calculated by constructing an archform that fits the majority of the teeth (Figure 35.1). Once the best fit of archform is chosen, it is then measured. Measurement of the archform is achieved by floss being placed around the constructed archwire, then measuring the floss. After the archform has been measured, measurement of the mesiodistal widths of all the teeth is required.

The total of the mesiodistal widths is then taken away from the total length of the constructed archform:

$$\text{Mesiodistal widths} - \text{Constructed archform} = \text{Total amount of crowding}$$

This is done for both upper and lower arches.

Crowding is classified as:

- Mild (<4 mm)
- Moderate (4–8 mm)
- Severe (>8 mm).

Previously clinicians would feed floss around the archform including displacements and measure the length of the floss, then compare this to a normal archform.

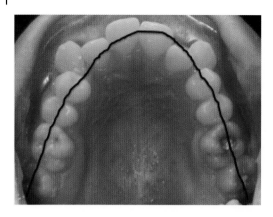

Figure 35.1 Assessing dental crowding.

35.2 Incisor Antero-posterior Change

When reduction of an overjet is needed, movement of the upper incisors changes, producing change in the AP position. When retraction is needed space is required, whereas when incisors are proclined space is gained. A normal overjet of 2 mm is the aim for every patient at the end of treatment; however, in some cases this may not be able to be the case.

In overjet reduction, achieving 1 mm of incisor retraction will require 2 mm of space within the dental arch. For example, if a patient presents with an overjet of 6 mm and the incisors need to be retracted to create a normal overjet of 2 mm, this would require space. Every 1 mm of incisor retraction requires 2 mm of space. So to reduce the overjet by 4 mm, the space required would be 8 mm.

35.3 Levelling Occlusal Curves

The curve of Spee is a curvature within the arch in the vertical dimension. When this requires levelling, space is needed. The amount of space varies, as the greater the depth of the curve the greater the space required. Dependent on the depth, the space required is indicated in Table 35.1.

When measuring the depth of the curve, the occlusal plane is drawn from the distal cusps of the first permanent molars to the incisors. The depth is then assessed from the premolar cusps to the occlusal plane (Figure 35.2).

Table 35.1 Space required to level the occlusal curve.

Depth	Space required
3 mm	1 mm
4 mm	1.5 mm
5 mm	2 mm

Figure 35.2 Space required to level the curve of Spee.

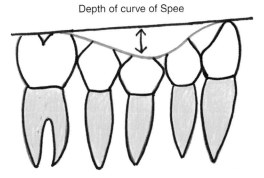

Depth of curve of Spee

35.4 Arch Expansion

Expansion of the dental arch can be an alternative way to create space. For expansion, for approximately every 1 mm of posterior arch expansion, 0.5 mm of space is gained. However, expansion should only be carried out if there is a crossbite present; if no crossbite is present this will increase the risk of instability and perforation of the buccal plate.

35.5 Creating Space

There are a number of ways in which space can be created:

- Extractions
- Distal movement of molars
- Enamel stripping
- Expansion
- Proclination of incisors
- A combination of any or all the above.

35.5.1 Extractions

Extractions are the most common technique used for creating space. First and second premolars are the most frequent teeth to be extracted. However, before these teeth are considered, if there are teeth with a poor prognosis these would be assessed first for extraction over a healthy tooth. Depending on where the area of crowding is, extractions should be done close to the site. For example, first premolars provide more space anteriorly than second premolars, therefore for crowding in the anterior region, first premolars would be considered.

35.5.1.1 Incisors

- Rarely extracted to create space.
- Only considered for extraction if:
  - They have poor prognosis.
  - Buccal segments are class I and there is lower incisor crowding.
  - There is a skeletal III pattern, as this helps to bring the lower incisors back.

35.5.1.2 Canines
Canines form the cornerstone of the arch and produce important aesthetic and functional factors, such as canine guidance for lateral movements. Extraction of these teeth is considered if:
- They are severely displaced, ectopic, or in an unfavourable position if impacted.
- There is a reasonable contact point between the lateral incisor and first premolar.

35.5.1.3 First Premolars
These teeth are the most common teeth be extracted and are considered if:
- There is the possibility of spontaneous alignment occurring.
- Moderate–severe crowding is present.

35.5.1.4 Second Premolars
These teeth are another common tooth/teeth to be extracted and are considered if:
- Mild–moderate crowding is present.
- Space closure is needed by forward movement of the posterior segment.
- There is severe displacement of the second premolar.

35.5.1.5 First Permanent Molars
Considered for extraction if there is a poor prognosis.

35.5.1.6 Second Permanent Molars
These teeth are considered for extraction if:
- Distal movement is needed in the upper buccal segments.
- There is a need to create space to relieve mild lower premolar crowding.
- There is a need to create additional space for eruption of third permanent molars.

35.5.1.7 Third Permanent Molars
Extraction of these teeth is considered if they are impacted or causing damage to other adjacent teeth, such as the second permanent molars.

35.5.2 Distal Movement of Molars

Headgear can be used to help achieve distalisation of the molars. Extra-oral traction can produce up to 2–3 mm of movement per side for a total of 4–6 mm of space.

35.5.3 Enamel Stripping

35.5.3.1 Interproximal Reduction
Sometimes interproximal reduction (IPR) is needed to create space. This involves the removal of a small amount of enamel between the mesial and distal aspects of the teeth. By doing this, space is created between the contact points to allow tooth movement to be achieved. It has also been known not just to create space, but to improve the shape and contact points of the teeth and enhance stability at the end of treatment. Removal of the enamel is achieved by an abrasive strip and approximately 0.5 mm can be removed on each tooth, which would be 0.25 mm on both the mesial and distal sides of that tooth.

35.5.3.2 Air-Rotor Stripping

This type of technique for removing enamel is the most common approach. A high-speed air-turbine handpiece is used which can create an additional 3–6 mm or more of space within the arch, as opposed to using an abrasive strip. The disadvantage of this approach is that it can cause damage to both the teeth and the periodontium.

35.5.4 Expansion

Creating space by use of arch expansion is another method. As mentioned earlier, expansion should only be used if a crossbite is present, therefore if a case presents with a crossbite, space can be achieved by expanding the arches. For every 1 mm of posterior expansion created, 0.5 mm of space is gained. Lower arch expansion is considered with cases that present with a lingual crossbite.

35.5.5 Proclination of Incisors

Creating space can be achieved by proclination of the incisors. Each 1 mm of incisor proclination creates approximately 2 mm of space within the dental arch.

36

Cleft Lip and Palate

Cleft lip and palate (CLP) is a cranio-facial malformation that is very common. It occurs in babies when the palatal horizontal process does not develop and fails to fuse together at eight weeks in the uterus.

There are two different types:

- Cleft lip with or without cleft palate.
- Isolated cleft palate.

36.1   Prevalence of Cleft Lip With or Without Cleft Palate

In Caucasians:

- Occurs in 1: 750 (with cleft palate) or 1: 1000 live births (without cleft palate).
- Males affected more than females at a ratio of 2: 1.
- The left side is the more commonly affected than the right.

36.2   Prevalence of Isolated Cleft Palate

In Caucasians:

- Occurs in 1: 200 live births.
- Females more affected than males at a ratio of 4: 1.

36.3   Syndromes Associated with Isolated Cleft Palate

The following are associated with isolated cleft palate:

- Down's syndrome
- Treacher Collins syndrome
- Pierre Robin syndrome
- Klippel–Feil syndrome.

Textbook for Orthodontic Therapists, First Edition. Ceri Davies.
© 2020 John Wiley & Sons Ltd. Published 2020 by John Wiley & Sons Ltd.

36.4 Aetiology

The cause of CLP can be multifactorial, with a combination of the following:

- *Genetic factors:* it could be passed on through the genes if there is a family history of CLP.
  Environmental factors: if during pregnancy the following supplements or drugs are taken this can increase the risk:
  – Vitamin A
  – Heroin
  – Anticonvulsant drugs
  – Steroids.
- As part of the syndromes listed previously.
- Folic acid deficiency during pregnancy can be a contributing factor, and is addressed with supplements for all pregnant women.

36.5 Development of CLP

Development of the hard and soft palate begins from two shelves that initially lie vertical on each side of the tongue. At eight weeks in the uterus, the tongue will lower, allowing the shelves to elevate vertically and then to join horizontally at the mid-palatine suture, where they will then fuse together. If the tongue does not drop this can result in the shelves not being able to fuse at the mid-palatine suture, therefore resulting in a cleft of the palate.

Failure of fusion can lead to either:

- Cleft of the lip and/or alveolus:
  – Unilateral (one side only).
  – Bilateral (both sides).
- Cleft of the lip and palate:
  – Unilateral (one side only).
  – Bilateral (both sides).

36.6 Classifications of CLP

There are three different classifications of CLP (Figure 36.1):

- *Primary palate – lip and alveolus:* the primary palate is located in front of the incisive foramen and can be affected by clefting of the lip and alveolus. It can affect one side (unilateral) or both sides (bilateral). In unilateral cases of clefting of the lip and alveolus, the base of the nose is flattened, with a deviation to the non-cleft side.
- *Cleft of the lip and palate:* cleft of the lip and palate can be unilateral or bilateral and present as complete or incomplete. Cases where there is a cleft of the lip and palate tend to have a small segment of alveolus move palatally and collapse inwards. Plastic surgeons and orthodontists can have problems aligning teeth in cases like this.
- *Cleft palate only:* clefting of the palate only affects the secondary palate. The soft palate may have a cleft, but this can extend to the hard palate too.

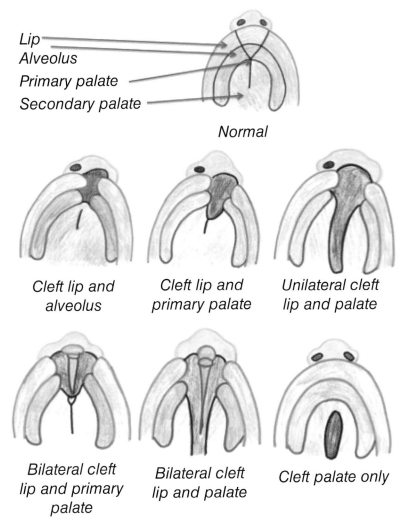

Lip
Alveolus
Primary palate
Secondary palate

Normal

Cleft lip and alveolus

Cleft lip and primary palate

Unilateral cleft lip and palate

Bilateral cleft lip and primary palate

Bilateral cleft lip and palate

Cleft palate only

Figure 36.1 Different types of cleft lip and palate.

36.7 Clinical Problems in CLP

There are many clinical problems that can arise from patients with CLP, which depend on the severity and location of the cleft. The following problems can be seen:

- *Feeding*: babies born with a CLP find it hard to achieve an oral seal.
- *Hearing*: a cleft in the posterior part of the hard and soft palate can affect hearing.
- *Speech*: the cleft can result in the soft palate being unable to make contact with the pharynx to close off the nasal airway, making speech difficult.
- *Dental anomalies*: a CLP affects the dentition and can result in:
  - Hypodontia
  - Supernumeraries

- Maxillary canine impaction
- Delayed dental development
- Hypoplastic teeth
- Microdontia
- Impaction of first permanent molars.
- *Malocclusion*: anterior and posterior crossbites can be present.
- *Deficient maxillary growth*: growth of the maxilla can be affected due to scarring of the maxilla following palate repair.
- *Low self-esteem*: patients can present with low self-esteem due to not feeling confident in the way they look because of the CLP.

36.8   CLP Team

Babies who are born with a CLP undergo treatment by the CLP team. These are experienced clinical experts who specialise in this condition. The team is made up of:

- Orthodontist
- Maxillofacial surgeon
- Plastic surgeon
- ENT surgeon – ears, nose, and throat
- Speech therapist
- Specialist health visitor.

36.9   Management of CLP

The CLP team will monitor each child's progress from birth until they stop growing at the age of 18 . Management involves a multidisciplinary approach for every patient:

- *Birth*
  - Visit from specialist health visitor
  - Rosti bottles to help with feeding.
- *Lip repair*
  - At 6–12 weeks of age muscle fibres are realigned.
- *Palate repair*
  - At 6–12 months of age, development of normal speech is encouraged.
- *Speech therapist*
  - Therapists help to encourage good speech and to detect any speech abnormality.
- *Further surgery*
  - Before the age of 4–5 years, further surgery may be considered to improve appearance before the child starts school.
- *Orthodontic care*

36.10   Orthodontic Implications of CLP

The following conditions can be seen in patients who were born with a CLP:

- Hypodontia, most commonly of upper lateral incisors
- Supernumeraries, most commonly the upper lateral incisor region

- Tooth pathology:
  - Abnormal size and shape
  - Enamel hypoplasia – enamel defect
  - Ectopic eruption of 6s.
- Crossbites
- Rotations
- Archforms
- Bone defects
- Class III malocclusions.

37

Orthognathic Surgery

37.1 Definitions

- *Orthognathic surgery* is specialist maxillofacial surgery. It works on realigning the jaws to improve the function and appearance.
- *Dentofacial deformity* is a deformity of the dentition and arch relationships, causing a deviation of the upper or lower jaws and resulting in the patient having difficulty in function due to aesthetics or jaw problems.

37.2 Indications for Treatment

Surgery is commonly used in patients who present with any of the following within the three planes of space:

- Antero-posterior dimension:
  - Severe class II skeletal discrepancies
  - Severe class III skeletal discrepancies.
- Vertical dimension:
  - Severe anterior openbite (AOB)
  - Severe deepbites.
- Transverse dimension:
  - Skeletal asymmetries.

37.3 Radiographs

Before surgery is considered, the relevant radiographs need to be taken to assess the patient:

- Dental panoramic tomography (DPT).
- Cephalometric radiograph and ceph analysis: this will help give detailed information about the relationships between different parts of the dentofacial complex, such as:
  - Cranium and cranial base
  - Naso-maxillary complex
  - Mandible
  - Maxillary and mandibular dentition.
- Upper standard occlusal.

Textbook for Orthodontic Therapists, First Edition. Ceri Davies.
© 2020 John Wiley & Sons Ltd. Published 2020 by John Wiley & Sons Ltd.

37.4 Surgical Procedures

There are many different surgical procedures that can be done, although every surgeon has their individual preference. The intra-oral approach is preferred as this avoids external scarring. There are different procedures for the maxilla and the mandible.

37.4.1 Maxillary Procedures

There are five different procedures that can be used on the maxilla, all to correct specific features.

37.4.1.1 Segmental Procedures

A maxillary segmental procedure involves moving the pre-maxilla region as a whole block, including the supporting bone structure. The term block of teeth refers to the canines and incisors as a whole unit. The intra-oral photograph in Figure 37.1 shows the segment that is moved after incisions have been made. The segment of teeth can be moved back to reduce an increased overjet or upwards to reduce an overbite.

This procedure still carries risks, such as increased morbidity due to tooth damage or reduced blood supply to the segment as a whole. Damage to the inferior orbital nerve can result in numbness to the cheek, upper lip, and side of the nose.

37.4.1.2 Le Fort I

Le Fort I is the most common maxillary procedure, and involves a horseshoe incision in the buccal mucosa and bone, freeing the maxilla. Once the maxilla is freed, only the palatal vessels and soft tissues are attached to it. With this incision the maxilla can then be moved to achieve correction for the following:

- To reduce a deepbite the maxilla is moved upwards, resulting in the bone being removed to move the segment up.
- To reduce an anterior overbite (AOB) the maxilla is moved downwards, resulting in a bone graft being needed.
- To move the maxilla forwards due to maxilla retrognathia, a bone graft is needed.
- To move the maxilla backwards due to maxilla prognathia, bone is removed.

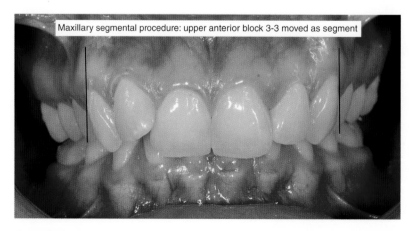

Maxillary segmental procedure: upper anterior block 3-3 moved as segment

Figure 37.1 Maxillary segmental procedure.

37.4.1.3 Le Fort II

Le Fort II covers a larger area than Le Fort I, as this surgery works to allow mid-face advancement. To enable correction of this, the nasal bones and zygomatic process are involved to permit movement. Surgical incisions can be done intra-orally or extra-orally. If using the intra-oral approach, the same process as Le Fort I is used. If the extra-oral approach is used, an incision is made in the infra-orbital region.

37.4.1.4 Le Fort III

Le Fort III is used when surgery is needed to correct any craniofacial anomalies. To achieve such a correction the bicoronal flap needs to be raised.

Figure 37.2 illustrates these three different types of segmental surgery: Le Fort I, II, and III.

37.4.1.5 Surgical Assisted Rapid Palatal Expansion

A surgical assisted rapid palatal expansion or SARPE (Figure 37.3) addresses transverse problems with the maxilla by achieving gradual widening by use of a rapid maxillary expander (RME). The RME is fitted by the use of molar bands connected onto the upper first premolars and molars, with rigid arms extended to the Hyrax screw. To achieve expansion, the surgeon splits the mid-palatine suture. After that the patient turns the key up to four times a day, resulting in 1 mm of movement per day. Once the maxilla has been widened sufficiently, the RME is left in situ for three months to

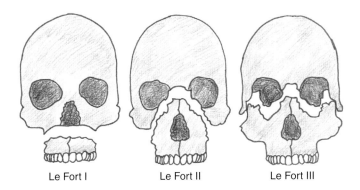

Le Fort I   Le Fort II   Le Fort III

Figure 37.2   Le Fort I, II, and III.

Figure 37.3   Surgical assisted rapid palatal expansion (SARPE).

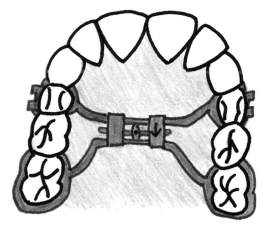

allow for the bony infill of the mid-palatine suture. Removal of the RME sooner than this can result in relapse.

A common feature seen with an RME is a diastema that will appear between the upper central incisors, which shows the results of the maxilla expanding.

37.4.2 Mandibular Procedures

There are six main types of surgery that can be used on the mandible, all to correct specific features.

37.4.2.1 Segmental Procedures

Segmental procedures are not only used on the maxilla, but also on the mandible (Figure 37.4). They work in a similar way to maxillary segmental procedures, by moving a block of teeth and their supporting bone and structures as a segment. Incisions again are made by the canines, including incisors, which are moved up or down depending on the type of case. Consideration of moving the segment down may be to reduce a deep overbite, whereas moving it up may be considered for cases presenting with an AOB.

The risk with this type of surgery is the increased mobility due to risk of tooth damage or reduced blood supply to the segment.

37.4.2.2 Vertical Subsigmoid Osteotomy

This type of surgery is used on mandibular retrognathic cases where the jaw needs to be brought forward. An incision is made down the ramus from the sigmoid notch to the lower border, which frees the bone, allowing the jaw to come forward (Figure 37.5). Surgery can be performed intra-orally by using special instruments or extra-orally with standard instruments, although with scarring post-surgery.

The advantage of this procedure is that the risk of nerve damage is less likely to occur due to the approach taken.

37.4.2.3 Bilateral Sagittal Split Osteotomy

A bilateral sagittal split osteotomy or BSSO is the most common surgery done on the mandible. It is used on patients presenting with severe mandibular retrognathism and prognathism. In skeletal class II cases, a BSSO is used to achieve mandibular advancement, whereas in a skeletal class III case it is to achieve the opposite, mandibular push reduction. Incisions are made intra-orally only

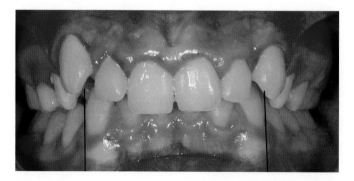

Figure 37.4 Mandibular segmental procedure.

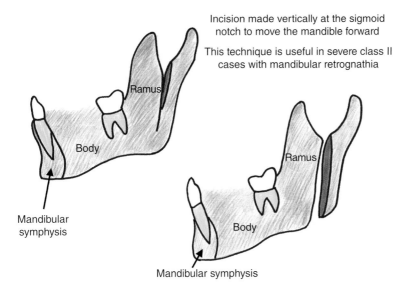

Figure 37.5 Vertical subsigmoid osteotomy.

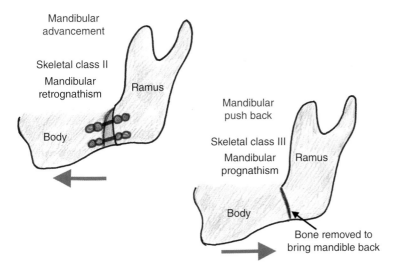

Figure 37.6 Bilateral sagittal split osteotomy.

behind the terminal molar directly into the buccal sulcus, with bony cuts made parallel across the angle of the mandible.

The risk of this surgery is that it can cause damage to the inferior dental nerve, which can lead to numbness and altered sensation to the lip and chin due to the mental nerve also being affected.

Figure 37.6 shows the involvement of the mandible for each case.

37.4.2.4 Body Osteotomy

A body osteotomy is rarely used nowadays, but is considered on patients who present with mandibular prognathism and have a natural gap in the lower arch anterior to the mental foramen (Figure 37.7).

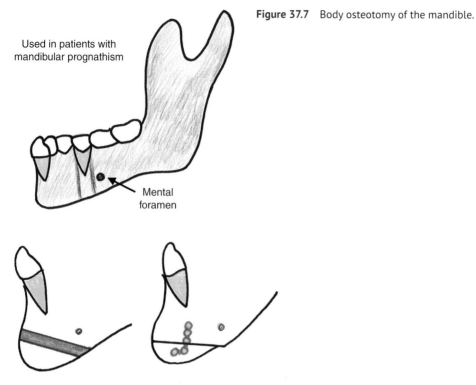

Figure 37.7   Body osteotomy of the mandible.

Used in patients with
mandibular prognathism

Mental
foramen

Figure 37.8   Where the incision is made for a genioplasty.

37.4.2.5   Genioplasty

A genioplasty is surgery performed on the chin (Figure 37.8). This type of surgery allows the chin to be moved in almost any direction, although this can be limited due to the sliding bony contact and muscle pedicle.

37.4.2.6   Post-Condylar Cartilage Graft

This type of surgery is used on actively growing patients with a severe mandibular retrognathia. Like functional appliance treatment, this surgery helps remodel the glenoid fossa by inserting a block of cadaveric or autologous cartilage behind the condylar head, producing an instant result.

37.4.3   Bimaxillary Surgery

In some cases both the maxilla and the mandible need to be moved. Bimaxillary surgery helps to correct an underlying skeletal discrepancy by repositioning both of these with screws.

37.4.4   Distraction Osteogenesis

This type of surgery is useful for correcting a severe deformity in growing children. It helps with the management of craniofacial anomalies and involves the application of incremental traction to osteotomised bone ends. By doing this it is hoped to help reduce the number of surgical procedures required.

37.5 Sequence of Treatment

Surgery cases include a sequence of treatment that is followed before the surgery itself.

37.5.1 Extractions

First in the sequence may be consideration of any extractions that may be needed. Extractions could be considered to help relieve crowding, level arches, and in some cases allow correction of the inclination of incisors, known as decompensation. Unerupted third permanent molars may also be considered for extraction prior to the start of treatment, as the surgeon may think these teeth could interfere with the planned surgery.

37.5.2 Pre-surgical Orthodontics

Before a patient has surgery, pre-surgical orthodontics is carried out to correct the following:

- Alignment and levelling
- Arch coordination
- Decompensation
- Creation of space for cuts
- Levelling and maintain the curve of Spee

Pre-surgical orthodontics is always carried out by the use of fixed appliances, which make it easier to attach intermaxillary elastics and obtain good correction of the incisors in the antero-posterior and vertical dimensions. The main aim of this prior to surgery is to allow for decompensation of the teeth by correcting the angulation of the incisors. This can make the patient look worse, as the full extent of the skeletal discrepancy becomes clear. It is important to ensure that the patient is aware of this and to reassure them that this is only temporary until the surgery is complete.

The overall process should take around 12–18 months and once completed a full new set of records are needed, such as impressions, photographs, and radiographs. This is to ensure that movements have been achieved ready for surgery.

37.5.3 Surgery

Surgery is done at the hospital, which involves a stay of two to four days. Small titanium plates and screws are used to hold the jaws in the new position. With the new jaws in this position, they are then closed down together by the use of intermaxillary fixation. Because the jaws are closed together, post-surgery liquid food is considered for the first few days, followed by a gradual increase from soft food to normal over a period of four to six weeks. Immediately after the operation the patient will be swollen; the swelling will go down rapidly during the first two to three weeks and reduce even more slowly over the next six to nine months.

Each approach to surgery can come with complications. Nerve damage, swelling, and bruising can occur to anyone who undergoes orthognathic surgery. It is important to ensure that the patient is aware of these complications prior to surgery being undertaken. If damaged, the infra-orbital nerve in the maxilla can result in numbness or altered sensation over the affected cheek and side of the nose. In the mandible, damage to the inferior dental nerve can also lead to numbness and altered sensation over the affected side of the chin and lip.

37.5.4 Post-surgical Orthodontics

Once surgery has been completed and the patient has fully recovered, orthodontic treatment can be completed. The aim of the post-surgical orthodontics is to achieve the following:

- Complete any movements not undertaken with pre-surgery orthodontics.
- Maintain surgical correction.
- Root paralleling at any segmental sites.
- Detailing and settling of occlusion.
- Inter-arch elastics on flexible wires to aid in settling.

37.6 Risks and Benefits

Orthognathic surgery comes with the risks and benefits.
   Risks:

- Discomfort – swelling, bruising, and pain post-surgery
- Loss/altered nerve sensation
- Reduced jaw function
- Infection
- Relapse.

   Benefits:

- Improvement in function
- Improvement in appearance
- Increase in self-esteem.

38

Retention and Stability

38.1 Definitions

- *Retention* is used to minimise relapse and maintain the result achieved at the end of treatment.
- *Relapse* is the return of teeth to the pre-treatment position from the result achieved from orthodontic treatment.

38.2 Aetiology of Relapse

There are four reasons why relapse can occur:

- Gingival and periodontal fibres
- Occlusal factors
- Soft tissue factors
- Growth factors.

38.2.1 Gingival and Periodontal Fibres

During tooth movement the periodontal ligaments are stretched, allowing the tooth to move through the alveolar bone. Due to the periodontium being stretched, the fibres within the ligament have a tendency to pull a tooth back to its original position until it adapts to its new location. Rotated teeth have a high tendency to relapse due to the movement needed to derotate them causing the periodontal ligament to stretch even further. It is important to ensure at the end of active treatment that the teeth are to be held long enough in their new position to reduce the possibility of relapse and increase their stability.

As well as holding the teeth in the correct position for longer in fixed appliance treatment, an alternative approach can be considered where the interdental and dento-gingival fibres can actively be cut, known as pericision.

Post-active treatment the alveolar bone and different fibres all take various amounts of time to settle down (Figure 38.1):

- Alveolar bone remodels within a month.
- Periodontal fibres rearrange in three to four months.

Textbook for Orthodontic Therapists, First Edition. Ceri Davies.
© 2020 John Wiley & Sons Ltd. Published 2020 by John Wiley & Sons Ltd.

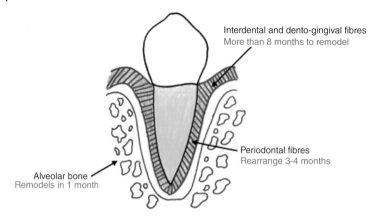

Figure 38.1 Gingival and periodontal fibres.

- Collagen fibres in the gingivae reorganise after four to six months.
- Elastic fibres in the dento-gingival and interdental fibres can take more than eight months to remodel.

38.2.2 Occlusal Factors

Correction is important after orthodontic treatment, as it can help prevent any relapse. Cases with a poorly finished occlusion can result in relapse, so it is important that the teeth occlude at the end of treatment. Good interdigitation at the end of treatment is likely to be more stable, for example teeth that are not fully interdigitated can result in the tongue thrusting between the teeth. This pressure can result in relapse, causing posterior and anterior openbites.

There are two methods which have been known to help with stability of the teeth at the end of treatment:

- As seen in Figure 38.2, stability is increased if the lower incisor edge lies 0–2 mm anterior to the mid-point of the root axis of the upper incisor, known as the centroid.
- A favourable interincisal angle of 135° or close to it produces a strong occlusal stop and prevents the incisors erupting past each other.

There is only one occasion where retainers are not needed and this is following correction of an anterior crossbite in interceptive treatment. This is because the correction of the crossbite is maintained by the overbite.

38.2.3 Soft Tissue Factors

The neutral zone is an area in which the teeth are situated between the tongue, cheeks, and lips. The tongue is the strongest soft tissue that can have an effect on the dentition. Because of the force it applies it is important to ensure, at the end of treatment, that the teeth are in the neutral zone, as this will increase stability. As an example in a class II div I case, when retracting the upper incisors back it is important to ensure that they fall under the control of the lower lip and tongue to reduce the risk of relapse. If teeth move out of the neutral zone, then there is a higher risk of

Figure 38.2 Correct centroid relationship.

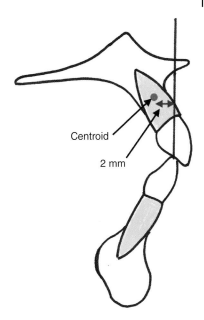

Centroid

2 mm

relapse. Providing the periodontium is healthy, the teeth will be maintained in a position of equilibrium.

There are two major problems with the neutral zone: first, nobody knows precisely where it is and how big it is; and second, due to the change in muscle tone as we get older, the neutral zone can change with age.

38.2.4 Growth Factors

Growth of a human is completed by the end of puberty. However, small changes can occur throughout life, which can have an effect on the positions of the maxilla and the mandible, resulting in the oral environment and pressures on the dentition constantly altering. If the pressures on the teeth are always changing, this can result in a high risk of relapse to the dentition as the patient gets older. An example of late growth changes can be seen when there is late lower incisor crowding in patients, whether or not they have had orthodontic treatment.

38.3 How Common Is Relapse?

The possibility of relapse cannot be identified in patients, making it unknown who will and who will not experience it. Therefore, all patients should be treated as if they could have potential relapse. Studies of relapse following fixed appliance treatment have shown that 10 years after retainers have been stopped, 70% of patients may need retreatment because of relapse occurring. Every 10 years the degree relapse continues to get worse. As it is not known who will and who will not experience relapse, patients who forget, or refuse, to wear retainers may be lucky enough to have no relapse at all, while others who have been compliant may suffer it.

38.4   Informed Consent for Retention

Prior to the start of orthodontic treatment, all patients must be informed about relapse and retention as part of informed consent, as commitment is required from the patient after the active treatment is completed. Every patient needs to be informed that they have the potential to relapse.

38.5   Retainers

Retainers are used to help reduce relapse and maintain the outcome achieved. It is important to ensure that the correct retention regimen is chosen for each individual patient. When choosing this, the following factors should be considered:

- Likely stability of the result
- Initial malocclusion
- Type of appliances used
- Oral hygiene
- Quality of result (any settling of occlusion required?)
- Compliance of patient
- Patient expectations
- Patient preference.

Retainers can come in two forms, removable or fixed. Each type has its own risks and benefits.

38.5.1   Removable Retainers

Patients are responsible for ensuring that these retainers are worn and, if they are not worn, the consequences that can arise and which they will have to accept. The benefit of having a removable retainer is that it facilitates good oral hygiene, since it can be removed for cleaning. Retainers are also capable of being worn part time if required, and from a clinical point of view it is the responsibility of the patient to ensure they are worn as instructed to prevent any relapse.

38.5.2   Fixed Retainers

This type of retainer is fixed to the teeth and cannot be removed by the patient. In some cases stability post-treatment can be extremely poor, therefore a fixed retainer may be required to prevent any relapse. Cases such as a diastema pre-treatment, correction of rotated teeth, substantial movement of the lower labial segment, and a lack of periodontal support all require fixed retainers for extra stability. However, as well as having a fixed retainer, since these to do not maintain stability to all of the teeth, the patient's care will be backed up with a removable retainer. This is known as dual retention. The advantages of fixed retainers are that they are useful when the end result is unstable and that the patient does not need to remember to wear them due to them being fixed to the teeth. The disadvantage of fixed retainers is that if they come loose, it is the responsibility of the clinician to put them back.

38.6 Removable Retainers

There are many types of removable retainers that can be used, including:

- Hawley
- Vacuum-formed
- Begg
- Barrier.

38.6.1 Hawley Retainer

A Hawley retainer (Figures 38.3 and 38.4) is a type of removable retainer that is used after orthodontic treatment, to maintain the end result and prevent any relapse. It is a simple robust appliance, which contains a labial bow, Adams clasps and an acrylic baseplate. In hypodontia cases prosthetic teeth can be added to the Hawley, although it is important to ensure that rigid stops are put on the retainer mesially and distally to prevent any relapse.

One of the advantages of this retainer is that it allows more rapid vertical occlusal settling of the teeth than vacuum-formed retainers because of its increased complete occlusal coverage.

A Hawley retainer is worn full time for three to six months, then nights only after that.

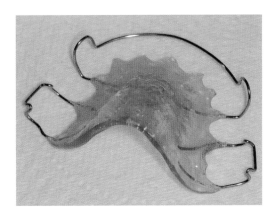

Figure 38.3 Hawley retainer.

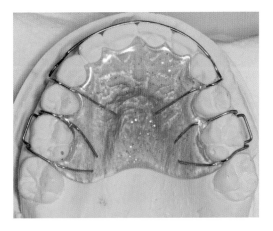

Figure 38.4 Hawley retainer, occlusal view.

The Hawley retainer can be modified with the addition of:

- *Acrylated labial bow*: a labial bow with acrylic facing. This gives more control of rotated teeth to prevent relapse.
- *Reverse U-loop*: this gives control to the canine position.
- *Passive flat anterior bite plane* (FABP): to maintain deep overbite correction.
- *Labial bow* soldered to clasps, so the wires do not interfere with occlusion.

Advantages:

- Simple to construct.
- Robust.
- Rigid enough to maintain transverse corrections.
- Easy to add prosthetic tooth.
- Can be worn for eating.
- Can help posterior occlusal settling.
- An anterior bite plane can be incorporated to help maintain overbite correction.
- The labial bow can be used for simple incisor tooth movement.

Disadvantages:

- Difficult for patients to tolerate, particularly lower.
- Expensive compared to vacuum-formed retainers.
- Can take time to make.

38.6.2 Vacuum-Formed Retainer

A vacuum-formed retainer (Figures 38.5 and 38.6) is a clear aligner that fits over the teeth to maintain the end result and prevent relapse. It has many potential advantages over a Hawley retainer. This type of retainer is worn full time for two days, being removed for eating and drinking anything other than water, then worn for nights only after that. Any other drinks such as cariogenic drinks must not be consumed with the retainer in place, as the retainer attracts the cariogenic liquid, which then will lay in contact with the incisal edges and cuspal tips, leading to decalcification, especially the upper retainer as this acts as a reservoir.

One disadvantage of this retainer is that the plastic can change the undercut gingival to the contact point, which can result to poor oral hygiene and cause hyperplastic gingivae.

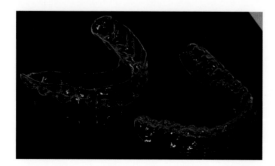

Figure 38.5 Vacuum-formed retainers.

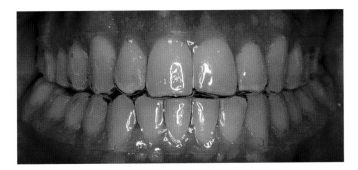

Figure 38.6 Vacuum-formed retainers in situ.

Advantages:

- Good aesthetics.
- Less interference with speech.
- More economical to make.
- Ease of fabrication.
- Superior retention of the lower incisors – better at preventing relapse.
- Preferred by patients.

Disadvantages:

- Can stop posterior occlusal settling.
- Not very durable – may need replacing.
- Need to cover the second molars to stop overeruption.

38.6.3 Begg Retainer

A Begg retainer (Figures 38.7 and 38.8) is considered if final settling of the occlusion and tooth positions is required. The retainer consists of a labial bow with adjustment loops at the canines, which extends closely and is contoured to the second permanent molars. Full-time wear of the retainer is required while the occlusion is settling, but once complete it is then worn nights only.

38.6.4 Barrier Retainer

A barrier retainer (Figure 38.9) is designed to allow minor adjustments to rotated incisors. As well as adjustment to incisors, it also allows for final settling of the occlusion, although this is for premolars only. The retainer is worn full time during adjustments, then once these are corrected it is worn every single night.

38.7 Fixed Retainers

Fixed retainers are attached to the palatal and lingual surfaces of the upper and lower anterior segments. They are bonded to the teeth using the normal acid-etch technique followed with composite bonding.

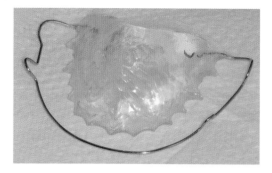

Figure 38.7 Begg retainer.

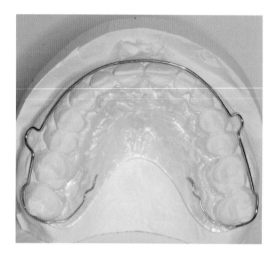

Figure 38.8 Begg retainer, occlusal view.

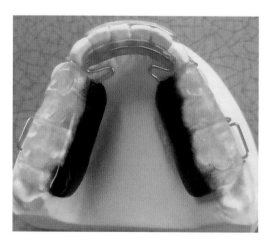

Figure 38.9 Barrier retainer.

There are five different types of fixed retainers:

- Multi-stranded retainers (Figure 38.10): bonded to each tooth 3–3, most commonly made of 0.0175 in. multi-stranded stainless-steel wire.
- Rigid bar (Figure 38.11): extending from canine to canine, but only bonded on the canines. This can result in relapse of the incisors.

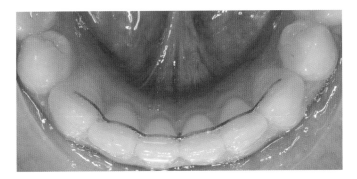

Figure 38.10 Multi-stranded fixed retainer.

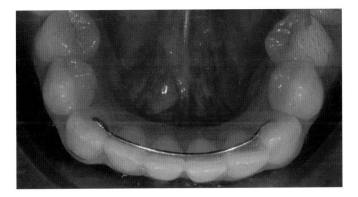

Figure 38.11 Rigid bar fixed retainer.

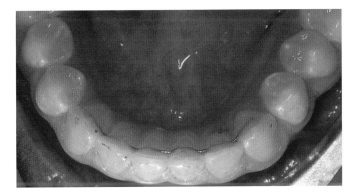

Figure 38.12 Preformed fixed retainer.

- Preformed fixed retainers (Figure 38.12).
- Custom-made retainers, either made chairside or at the laboratory.
- Reinforced fibre retainers.

Placement of a fixed retainer requires a good technique. The tooth surface must be clear of any calculus that could be present, as this can result in failure of bonding, and the area must be dry and well maintained. On bonding the acid-etch technique is used and the wire is held passively in position against the teeth while composite is used to bond to the teeth. Failure of bonding to the teeth can result in relapse even if the fixed retainer is partially debonded.

Patients who have a fixed retainer will be supplied with a removable retainer too, which is known as dual retention. This can help prevent any relapse of the teeth if the fixed retainers are to debond away. Backing up with a removable retainer at night will not only help prevent relapse if the fixed retainer has debonded away, but will prevent relapse of posterior teeth. Patients are to be seen on a regular basis for any bond failures.

Fixed retainers are usually used for specific problems:

- Correction of rotations.
- Mid-line diastema.
- Generalised spacing.
- Severely displaced teeth.
- Periodontal problems.

Advantages:

- Discreet – good aesthetics.
- Reduced demands on patient compliance.

Disadvantages:

- High failure rate.
- Oral hygiene is difficult.
- Requires long-term maintenance.

38.8   Care of Removable and Fixed Retainers

Each type of retainer involves different cleaning methods:
   Removable retainers:

- Easier to care for – removed for oral hygiene.
- Toothbrush and toothpaste – acrylic-based retainers.
- Special cleaning materials such as Retainer Brite for cleaning vacuum-formed retainers that do not degrade the plastic.

   Fixed retainers:

- Potential to cause periodontal disease and caries unless well maintained.
- Clean interdentally by floss threaded under wire or with small interdental brushes.

38.9   Enhancing Stability

There are two techniques that can be considered to help enhance stability: pericision and enamel interproximal stripping.

- The pericision technique is known as circumferential supracrestal fiberotomy. This procedure involves cutting the interdental and dento-gingival fibres above the alveolar bone. These fibres have a tendency to pull teeth back into their original position, especially on teeth that have been severely rotated. The procedure is undertaken with local anaesthetic and requires no periodontal

dressings after the cuts are made. The cuts are made vertically into the periodontal pocket, severing fibres around the neck of the teeth not touching the alveolar bone. This procedure can reduce relapse by up to 30% and is most effective in the maxilla.
- Enamel interproximal stripping is also known as reproximation and involves removal of small amounts of enamel mesio-distally. Doing this reshapes teeth and creates small amounts of space between the teeth. It has been suggested that flattening the interdental contact increases the stability between the adjacent teeth.

38.10   Types of Tooth Movement to Be Retained

The following types of tooth movement all need retaining with the use of retainers:

- Tipping
- Bodily movement
- Rotation
- Intrusion
- Extrusion.

38.11   General Advice on Retention

- Night-time wear forever (for however long the patient wants straight teeth!).
- Retainers must be worn 10–12 hours per night.

38.12   Five Key Points

1) Relapse is unpredictable.
2) Relapse can be due to orthodontic factors.
3) Relapse can be due to unfavourable growth.
4) Relapse and retention must be part of the informed consent process.
5) Patient must recognise their responsibility in the retention phase.

38.13   Outcome and Follow-Up After Debonding

- Retention appointments are required after debonding.
- When retention is stable, the patient can be discharged from routine appointments.
- All appropriate information must be given prior to discharge:
  - Maintenance and care of retainers including replacement costs.
  - Need to continue long-term retention.
- Continue regular general dental check-ups.
- Return to orthodontist if concerned about retainers or tooth alignment.
- All patient records stored and archived indefinitely.

39

Interceptive Treatment

39.1 Definition

Interceptive treatment is also known as early treatment and is carried out in the early mixed dentition stage, from the age of 7 years. Early treatment may be considered to relieve any occlusal interference that has occurred during eruption. This manages the dentition by preventing unwanted interferences that can occur in the future once the remaining teeth have erupted. Situations in which interceptive treatment may be utilised are summarised in Table 39.1.

39.2 Clinical Interceptive Situations: Early Mixed Dentition

39.2.1 Increased Overjet

- Removable appliance incorporating a labial bow to retract upper incisors:
  - Used in patients with a good skeletal pattern but just needing retraction of the upper anterior segment.
- Functional appliances:
  - Used in patients with skeletal II patterns and an increased overjet.

39.2.2 Supernumerary Teeth

Any supernumerary teeth can be extracted if they post a high risk to the other permanent dentition, or they can be left alone and monitored.

39.2.3 Early Loss of Deciduous Teeth: Space Maintenance

When there is early loss of any deciduous teeth, a space maintainer may be used. Clinical situations where a space maintainer may be considered would be the following:
- Early loss of the second deciduous molars:
  - Mesial movement of the first permanent molar into the second deciduous molar space can result in impaction to the second premolar.
  - By maintaining space, this will allow normal eruption of the second premolar.

Textbook for Orthodontic Therapists, First Edition. Ceri Davies.
© 2020 John Wiley & Sons Ltd. Published 2020 by John Wiley & Sons Ltd.

Table 39.1 Clinical situations for interceptive treatment.

Clinical situations	
Early mixed dentition	• Increased overjet
	• Supernumerary teeth
	• Early loss of deciduous teeth
	• Delayed eruption of the maxillary central incisor
	• Impaction of first permanent molars
	• Anterior crossbites
	• Posterior crossbites
	• Severe crowding
	• Digit sucking habits
	• Severe crowding
Late mixed dentition	• Infraocclusion
	• Ectopic maxillary canines
	• Hypodontia
	• Traumatic overbites
	• Increased overjet
	• Poor-quality first permanent molars
Early permanent dentition	• Hypodontia
	• Crowding
	• Impacted teeth

- Early loss of the first deciduous molars before eruption of the first permanent molars:
  - Early loss of the first deciduous molars before eruption of the first permanent molars can result in mesial movement, leading to impaction of the first premolars.
- Loss of the deciduous canines on one side (unilateral):
  - If unilateral loss of a deciduous canine occurs, drifting of the remaining teeth within that arch can cause a centreline shift, leading to space loss for the permanent canine.
  There are various space-maintaining appliances that can be used.

39.2.3.1 Removable Appliance

- Upper removable appliance (URA) used for space maintenance to allow eruption of permanent teeth or for implants (Figure 39.1).
- Advantages:
  - Removed to enable the patient to maintain good oral hygiene.
  - Easy to adjust when permanent teeth erupt, for example removing acrylic when needed.
- Disadvantages:
  - Patient compliance, as if the appliance is not worn space closure can occur.
  - Can become loose over time.

39.2.3.2 Partial Denture (Pontic)

- Pontics allow for good aesthetics for missing tooth/teeth.
- Pontics also enable the patient's bite to function.
- As pontics help with the functioning of the patient's bite, this prevents overeruption of opposing teeth.

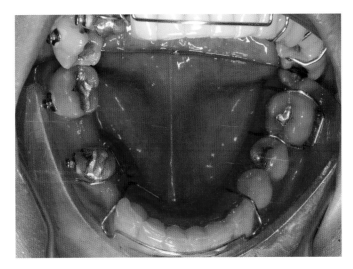

Figure 39.1 Occlusal view of a space maintainer which is being used to help distalise LR5 to make space for an implant. Retentive components are being used to maintain space while distalising.

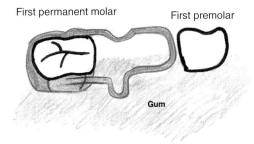

Figure 39.2 Band and loop being used for space maintenance. To prevent mesial movement of the first permanent molar, the extended loop is being maintained to keep the space so that passive eruption of the second premolar can be achieved.

- Advantages:
  - Good aesthetics for the patient.
  - Can be removed by the patient.
  - Improves patient's confidence.
- Disadvantages:
  - Patient compliance, as if pontic is not worn space closure can occur.
  - Can become loose over time.

39.2.3.3 Band and Loop

- Fixed space maintainer.
- Consists of a molar band and an extended stainless-steel arm with soldered loops.
- Used to prevent mesial movement of the first permanent molars due to early loss of the second deciduous molar.
- Extended arm sits from the molar band to the distal aspect of the first premolar, maintaining the space for eruption of the second premolar (Figure 39.2).

- Advantages:
  - Appliance is fixed to the teeth and cannot be removed by the patient.
  - Easy to place.
- Disadvantages:
  - Can be difficult to clean.
  - Requires more appointments prior to fit.

39.2.3.4 Distal Shoe

- Fixed space maintainer.
- Works in a similar way to the band and loop.
- Consists of a molar band with an extended stainless-steel arm that sits distal to the premolar 1 mm under the gingival margin (Figure 39.3).
- Used to prevent mesial movement of the first permanent molar due to early loss of the second deciduous molar.
- Advantages:
  - Appliance is fixed to the teeth and cannot be removed by the patient.
  - Less chance of space loss as opposed to a removable appliance when not worn.
- Disadvantage:
  - Hard to keep clean.
  - More appointments needed prior to fitting.

39.2.3.5 Lingual Arch

- Used as a fixed space maintainer on the lower arch only.
- Consists of lower molar bands with an extended stainless-steel arch that maintains arch length (Figure 39.4).
- Prevents mesial movement of the lower permanent molars when there is early loss of the lower second deciduous molars.
- Extended stainless-steel arch maintains lower anterior incisors, preventing them from retroclining.
- Advantages:
  - Appliance is fixed to the teeth and cannot be removed by the patient.

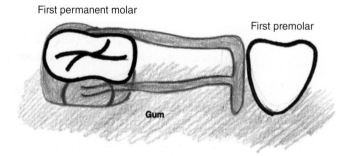

First permanent molar

First premolar

Gum

Figure 39.3   Distal shoe. This is similar to a band and loop, however the extension of the digital shoe is extended subgingivally 1 mm below the distal aspect of the first premolar, to prevent mesial movement of the first permanent molar.

Figure 39.4 Lingual arch.

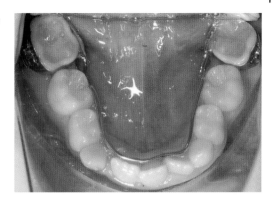

Figure 39.5 Transpalatal arch with Nance button.

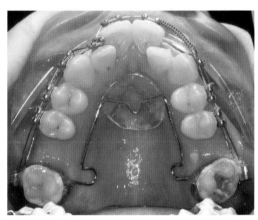

- Disadvantages:
  - Can be difficult to clean.
  - Requires more appointments prior to fitting.

39.2.3.6 Transpalatal Arch (TPA) with Nance Button

- Can be used as a fixed space maintainer as well as an anchorage device.
- Used in the upper arch only.
- Consists of molar bands on the upper first permanent molars, with extended stainless-steel arms that extend to the palatal vault, with an acrylic button incorporated that lies on the palatal mucosa (Figure 39.5).
- Helps to prevent mesial movement of the upper first molars through resistance from either the maxillary vault or basal bone, but mainly the maxillary vault.
- Pressure applied on the Nance button.
- Also prevents rotation to the upper first permanent molars.
- Advantages:
  - Fixed to the teeth and cannot be removed by the patient.
  - Not dependent on compliance by the patient.
- Disadvantages:
  - Difficult to clean.
  - Gingiva can form over acrylic Nance button when too much force is applied, resulting in embedding.

39.2.3.7 TPA

- Can be used as a fixed space maintainer as well as an anchorage device.
- Used in the upper arch only.
- Consists of molar bands on the upper first permanent molars, with 0.9 mm of stainless-steel arm that transverses the hard palate, connecting to each molar band (Figure 39.6).
- Stops the upper first permanent molars moving mesially, which is achieved as soon as the mesio-buccal root of the upper first permanent molar hits cortical bone.
- Extended arm also fixes the maxillary intermolar width, which helps to prevent these teeth from moving mesially.
- Advantages:
  - Fixed to the teeth and cannot be removed by the patient.
- Disadvantages:
  - Difficult to clean.
  - Can become dislodged due to too much force and embed in the palate.

39.2.4 Delayed Eruption of Maxillary Central Incisor

The maxillary central incisor should erupt at the age of 7 years. If there is no sign of eruption by the age of 8–9, observations should be made to establish why this tooth is delayed and treatment options considered to encourage eruption. Before any treatment is carried out, an upper standard occlusal or dental panoramic tomography (DPT) radiograph should be taken to determine if the maxillary central incisor is in a favourable position to come down. The following treatment options are considered:

- URA used for space maintainer:
  - If the tooth is in a favourable position to erupt, a URA can be used for space maintenance to maintain its space while encouraging eruption.
- Exposure if the tooth is impacted:
  - Removable appliance used after exposure to help bring the tooth down via gold chain if closed exposure or ligation by attachment, and some form of tie such as a metal ligature or zing string if an open exposure.
  - Sectional fixed appliance used after exposure to help bring the tooth down with the same form of attachment.

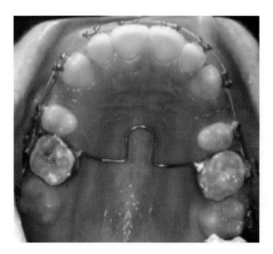

Figure 39.6 Transpalatal arch.

39.2.5 Impaction of First Permanent Molars

The first permanent molars erupt at the age of 6 years. If these teeth are unerupted, then further investigation is needed to locate where they are. Once appropriate radiographic examination has been done to locate these teeth, then the following steps should be considered:

- Observation:
  - This approach could be considered in cases where the first permanent molars are in a favourable position.
  - However, review may be considered in three to six months to see if there is any improvement.

If the teeth are in an unfavourable position (impacted or non-impacted):

- Separation:
  - Needed to move the first permanent molar distally.
  - Achieved by use of a metal separator known as a brass wire.
  - Inserted by the contact point of the mesial aspect of the first permanent molar.
  - Inserted by use of light wire pliers.
  - Tightened once a week to ensure equal force.
- URA:
  - With palatal finger springs incorporated to distalise the first permanent molars
- Fixed appliances:
  - With either TPA, TPA with Nance, or headgear.
  - Helps to achieve distalisation or move first permanent molars distally.
- Headgear:
  - Used to distalise first permanent molars.
- Extracting second deciduous molar:
  - Can be considered to help eruption of first permanent molar if root resorption of second deciduous molar is severe.
  - Disadvantage of this approach is that loss of space for the second premolars can occur, leading to future impaction of these teeth and crowding in this area.

39.2.6 Anterior Crossbite

To correct an anterior crossbite, a removable appliance is considered. This has incorporated an anterior expansion screw or Z springs with a posterior bite plane. Another option could be to use a sectional fixed appliance to correct the torque of the teeth, relieving them out of an anterior crossbite by the use of round and later rectangular archwires.

39.2.7 Posterior Crossbite

A posterior crossbite is seen when expansion of the upper arch is needed. There are four approaches that can be considered when correcting a posterior crossbite:

- Removable appliance incorporating a midline expansion screw or coffin spring with posterior bite planes:
  - Turned by a key once a week, a quarter turn of 0.25 mm.
- Rapid maxillary expansion (RME):
  - Should not be used after the age of 17–18 years as the mid-palatal suture becomes more fused at this age, so separation is less likely to happen.
  - Turned four times a day to produce 1 mm of expansion a day.

- Quadhelix:
  - Expands upper arch to correct posterior crossbites.
- Functional regulator appliance – Frankel:
  - Produces expansion by use of the buccal shields that are incorporated within the appliance.
  - These shields eliminate the cheek pressure by holding the soft tissues away from the dentition, allowing for the expansion to be achieved.

39.2.8   Severe Crowding

Early treatment may be considered if there is severe crowding in the mixed dentition stage. Spontaneous tooth movement can occur and crowding can correct itself, so it may be decided to observe and review the patient to see if the crowding does so. If it does not, a URA may be considered to make space for eruption of the other permanent dentition or to tip teeth into a better position by use of T springs and Z springs to make space within the arch.

39.2.9   Digit Sucking Habits

- A persistent digit sucking habit that the patient cannot stop means that persistent pressure from the thumb/finger can cause occlusal disruption to both upper and lower arches.
- If the habit has not stopped by the age of 7–8 years, a treatment approach to stop the habit is considered, especially when the upper central incisors, lateral incisors, and first permanent molars have erupted.
- Treatment approaches to stop the habit include:
  - Removable appliance with deterrent dissuader (habit breaker).
  - Fixed digit deterrent dissuader.
  - Quadhelix – can also be used as a habit breaker.

39.3   Clinical Situations: Late Mixed Dentition

39.3.1   Infraocclusion

Infraocclusion is where teeth erupt but their occlusal surface is below the adjacent teeth. When this is seen, it is most commonly because the tooth/teeth are ankylosed or submerged, meaning the tooth is fused to the bone and has no periodontal ligament. In such cases options are considered if the permanent tooth underneath is also missing (known as hypodontia). The following options are considered:

- Monitor the infraoccluded teeth:
  - If there are no occlusal interferences within the arch.
  - Considered only in mild cases.
- Restore the infraoccluded teeth:
  - Restoring the occlusal surfaces will help with:
    o Better functioning of the bite.
    o Preventing tipping of adjacent teeth.
    o Preventing overeruption of opposing teeth where they do not meet.

- Complete submergence of the teeth:
  - Extraction is considered alongside tipping of the adjacent teeth if seen.

39.3.2 Ectopic Maxillary Canines

- An ectopic canine is when a canine is not following its normal path of eruption within the maxilla.
- Ectopic canines can lead to impaction.
- Treatment options:
  - Observe by radiographs to review the position of the ectopic canine.
  - Extraction of the deciduous canine may be considered to help with eruption of the ectopic canine.
  - If no improvement within 12 months, alternative treatment can be considered such as appliances to expand the upper arch in both transverse and antero-posterior planes.
  - If still no improvement, exposure is needed to help bring the tooth down.

39.3.3 Hypodontia

- Missing teeth can cause psychological issues for the patient. If that occurs, a partial denture could be considered to improve the situation for early treatment.
- Microdontia is a common clinical sign that is associated with hypodontia, and if there is a build-up of these teeth there may be a need to reduce spacing.

39.3.4 Traumatic Overbites

- URA with flat anterior bite plane (FABP):
  - Allows passive lower molar eruptions and intrusion of the lower anterior segment.
  - Increases wedge effect to open the patient's bite.
- Clark's twin block appliance:
  - Used in patients with a skeletal class II.
  - Used to posture the mandible forward, causing stretching of the facial soft tissues and muscles to reduce an overjet.
  - Results in posterior openbites at the end of treatment.
  - Good for patients with deepbites, as appliance increases the vertical skeletal growth, opening the patient's bite.

39.3.5 Increased Overjet

- URA with active labial bow:
  - Used in patients with a good skeletal pattern, but just needing retraction of the upper anterior segment.
  - Activation of the labial bow can help to reduce overjet by retracting upper anterior segment.
- Functional appliances:
  - Used in patients with skeletal II patterns and an increased overjet.
  - Used to posture the mandible forward, causing stretching of the facial soft tissues and muscles to reduce an overjet.

39.3.6 Poor-Quality First Permanent Molars

- Enamel hypoplasia present on first permanent molars.
- Extraction of these teeth may be considered in severe cases.
- This will allow eruption of the second permanent molars to take their place and at a later date allow for the third permanent molars to erupt if present.

39.4 Clinical Situations: Early Permanent Dentition

39.4.1 Hypodontia

- Missing teeth.
- Fixed appliances.
- Leave opened space for prosthetics (implants, bridges).
- Close space (build up premolar to look like canine and canine to look like incisor).

39.4.2 Crowding

- Fixed appliances to relieve crowding.
- Possible extractions may be considered.

39.4.3 Impacted Teeth

- Open or closed exposure.
- Fixed appliances to help extrude and align impacted tooth.

39.5 Serial Extractions

This procedure was introduced in the 1940s and is rarely used today. It was used to treat class I malocclusions with severe crowding in the upper and lower labial segments. It was an alternative to orthodontic treatment, as it was believed that using this approach would help to align the dentition without the need for any type of orthodontic appliance.

Disadvantages:

- Can result in the procedures being done under general anaesthetic each time.
- Can be an unpleasant experience for the patient, making it stressful for them.
- Results in space loss due to mesial drift of adjacent teeth.
- Can lead to impaction of the first premolars if they have not erupted, as the lower canines could possibly erupt into the first premolar space, resulting in impaction of these teeth.
- Can only be done on class I malocclusions as it does not correct the anterio-posterior position of the incisors.
- Can cause the lower incisors to retrocline, which then can result in a deepbite.
- Risk of alignment not being achieved, resulting in the patient needing an orthodontic appliance to correct what should have been corrected by the procedure.
- Patient undergoes a lot of extractions.

The procedure for when and how serial extractions are undertaken is listed in Table 39.2. All together this is a total of 12 extractions the patient has to go through.

Table 39.2 Procedure for serial extractions.

Procedure	Notes
Extraction of four deciduous canines – Cs	• At approximately 8 years old on eruption of the maxillary lateral incisors • This will allow the upper incisors to align using the canine space
EXTRACTION OF THE FIRST DECIDUOUS MOLARS – Ds	• At approximately 9 years old when the roots of the successor are half formed • This is thought to help the first premolars to erupt before the canines
Extraction of the first permanent premolars – 4s	• This is done just before the permanent canines erupt, after confirmation that the canines are buccally placed and mesially angulated • This is only carried out if moderate to severe crowding is present

40

Adult Orthodontics

Orthodontic treatment is not just available for children under the age of 18 on the NHS, but can also be done privately for those who do not meet the Index of Orthodontic Treatment Need (IOTN) requirements and adult patients. Treatment for adults has increased and become more popular over the years. With there being many more options of different appliances available, adult patients are now not worried about having treatment, as there are appliances that can suit different life styles. Metal appliances are still available for patients who wish to have them, but as they are more aesthetically and socially pleasing, more adults want to have treatment.

40.1 Reasons for Adult Orthodontics

There could be many reasons for adults wanting treatment:

- *Dental aesthetics*: some adults may wish to improve their dental aesthetics, for instance to relieve crowding, improve the function of the bite, for space closure, and for reduction in an overjet.
- *Restorative treatment* (interdisciplinary case): a patient could need treatment from a range of professionals, such as:
  - *Implants*: orthodontic treatment would help to upright roots (root paralleling) of adjacent teeth to ensure there is enough space for placement of an implant. Average required space for an implant is 7 mm.
  - *Bridges*: space may need to be created or reduced to allow for restorative work of bridges to be done from missing teeth.
  - *Build-ups*: worn-down teeth may require build-ups once the teeth are aligned.
  - *Space closure*: due to failing restorations, closing gaps can result in reduced replacement of fillings.
- *Relapse*: some adults may have had treatment as a child, but not wearing retainers has caused their teeth to move back to the original position, leading to them wanting to have treatment again.

40.2 Differences in Treating Adult Patients

The biggest difference in treating an adult as opposed to a child is the treatment time, which is greatly increased due to many factors:

Textbook for Orthodontic Therapists, First Edition. Ceri Davies.
© 2020 John Wiley & Sons Ltd. Published 2020 by John Wiley & Sons Ltd.

- *Unfavourable growth*: movement of teeth is not as quick in non-growing patients.
- *Medical history*: adults tend to be on more medication than children, and some medication can have an effect on tooth movement by slowing the process down. It has been known that some hormone replacement therapy (HRT) medication that women take can have an effect on tooth movement as the bone firms up, making it difficult to achieve tooth movement.
- *Expectations*: adults may be more demanding to treat due to possibly having high expectations of what they wish to achieve. However, they may be more compliant than a child regarding the brace.
- *Reduced cellular activity*: due to reduced vascularity of the periodontal ligament, tooth movement can take longer and because of this more pain may be experienced from archwire adjustments. Greater root resorption may also be experienced.
- *Dental disease*: any previous dental disease can have an effect on treatment, such as periodontal disease, caries, tooth wear, missing teeth, and most importantly heavy restorations such as crowns, since bonding of brackets is not as efficient. No orthodontic treatment should be carried out on adult patients with active periodontal disease. Patients must be made fully aware that any periodontal disease must be under control first.
- *Periodontal ligament*: relapse is higher in an adult, as the ligament and fibres do not adapt to their new position as quickly, therefore retention in an adult should be increased.
- *Compromising treatment*: as adults are not growing some patients may require orthognathic surgery to correct their underlying skeletal problems. For example, for a patient with an increased overjet who requires orthognathic surgery for mandibular advancement, if the patient does not wish to have this done, compromising the overjet may have to be considered.

40.3 Aesthetic Appliances

Over the years many appliances have been developed and there is now a lot more choice for adult patients, with many aesthetically and socially pleasing options.

- *Clear buccal fixed appliances* are very popular today. Many adults like this brace as it is less noticeable and can be used with white, Teflon-coated wires (Figure 40.1).
- *Invisalign*® (Align Technology, San Jose, CA, USA) has become very popular over the years. This appliance allows patients to remove the brace at any time. To enable this appliance to work, patients have tooth-coloured attachments bonded to the teeth, helping to achieve tooth movement with the aligner in place. Invisalign now can be used on extraction cases and have intermaxillary elastic wear attached to it (Figure 40.2).
- *Lingual appliances* are fixed appliances bonded onto the lingual/palatal surfaces of the teeth (Figure 40.3). An advantage of this brace is that it is bonded on the inside of the teeth, making it unnoticeable. The disadvantage is that treatment time is increased and it is very hard to tolerate, especially on the lower arch, as it can cause irritation to the tongue.

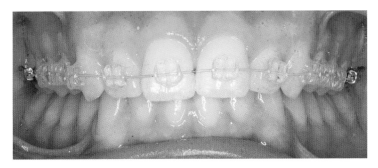

Figure 40.1 Aesthetic brackets (Spa, DB Orthodontics, Silsden, UK) with Teflon-coated archwire and clear modules.

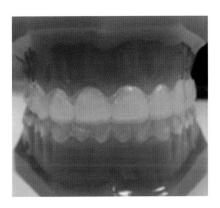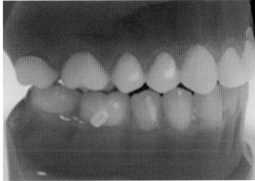

Figure 40.2 Invisalign model showing aligner, attachments, and composite buttons.

Figure 40.3 Lingual appliance.

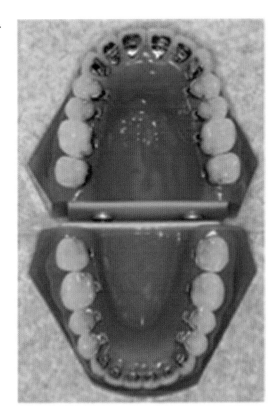

41

Orthodontic Materials

Many different materials are used in orthodontics. Each material helps to bond different appliances to the teeth, but all serve different purposes.

The following materials are in use:

- Etch
- Bond – adhesives
- Composites
- Cements

41.1   Etch

Etch is a phosphoric acid which comes in the form of a liquid or gel and is used to prepare the tooth surface for bonding of an orthodontic attachment.

Etch contains 20–40% phosphoric acid; however, the most commonly used today is 37%.

Etch that comes in a form of a gel is safer to use as it is more visible and easier to localise than a liquid form. No matter which type is used, etch must always be handled with care. Any part of it that makes contact with the mucosa or skin can cause burning, which will lead to permanent scarring.

41.1.1   Using Etch

Etch is used to help prepare a tooth surface for bonding of an orthodontic attachment. When the etch is applied to the tooth surface, it leaves exposed crystalline structures within the enamel (Figure 41.1). The pitted areas on the tooth surface enable the bond to flow between these structures, allowing for a *mechanical bond*. This is increased with the mesh base on the back of the brackets.

Once etch has been applied to the tooth, it is washed off and fully dried, giving it the frosty white look, and primer is then placed. The purpose of the primer is to allow penetration of the enamel surface, which helps to improve the effectiveness of the final bond. With the use of a microbrush the primer is rubbed onto the tooth surface for three seconds where the attachment is going to be placed, which will make the tooth shiny. Priming a tooth produces a *chemical bond*, which allows for polymerization, the process in which two molecules join together, sharing anatomical structures. If at any point during this stage saliva makes contact with the teeth, bonding of the attachment will fail and the etch will need to be reapplied.

Textbook for Orthodontic Therapists, First Edition. Ceri Davies.
© 2020 John Wiley & Sons Ltd. Published 2020 by John Wiley & Sons Ltd.

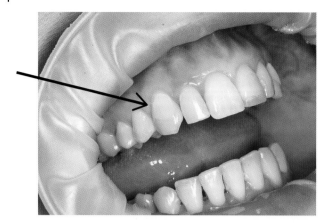

Figure 41.1 Exposed crystalline structures. Etch applied to the tooth (arrow) leaves exposed crystalline structures and makes teeth look frosty white.

There are two ways in which etch can be applied to a tooth: the acid etch technique and self-etch primer.

41.1.2   Acid Etch Technique (37% Phosphoric Acid)

The acid etch technique is a procedure that involves applying etch to the tooth surface and leaving it in placed for 20–30 seconds. After this time it is washed away with a three-in-one syringe (Figure 41.2) and fully dried in the air. Once fully dried, the primer is then placed on the tooth surface prior to bonding the orthodontic attachment with composite. This starts as a mechanical bond then progresses to a chemical bond. A gel etch and the process of mechanical and chemical bonds are illustrated in Figure 41.3).

41.1.3   Self-Etch Primer

Self-etch primer (SEP) comes in a liquid form known as a lollipop, which is etch and primer together (Figure 41.4). This combines the whole process into one, ready for composite placement,

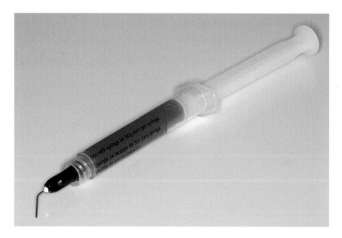

Figure 41.2 Phosphoric acid applicator.

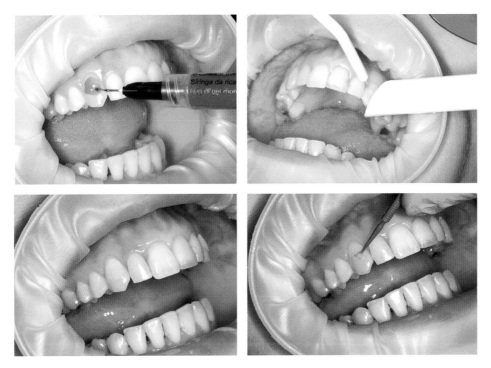

Figure 41.3 Acid etch technique procedure.

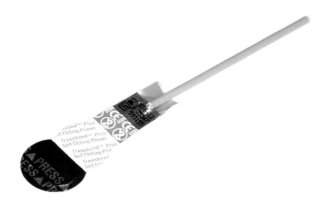

Figure 41.4 Self-etch primer.

so there is no need to prime after etching. Each lollipop contains phosphate monomers with a low pH and the acidity is neutralised by the release of Ca^{2+}. The biggest advantage of this process is that it is moisture tolerant, so if the tooth gets wet the orthodontic attachment will still bond to the tooth.

The SEP comes in a sheath:

- The black reservoir liquid is squeezed into the white reservoir, towards the disposable applicator, and then folded where it meets with the white reservoir to stop the liquid following back.
- White and back reservoir are then folded over each other and the liquid in the white reservoir is then squeezed into the purple reservoir onto a disposable applicator ready to use.

Once the SEP has been applied, the prism core and boundaries from the etch dissolve at different rates (differential dissolution), creating a porous surface. Achieving a porous surface will provide an opportunity for the cement to mechanically lock, making a micro-mechanical zip.

After the liquid enters the purple reservoir, it is then ready to be applied. By use of the microbrush the liquid is applied to the tooth surface and rubbed into the enamel. The liquid should be honey coloured on the applicator and should cover the correct area. Once applied gently, air dry the tooth/teeth so there is an even bond ready for the composite.

41.2 Adhesives

Adhesives are materials used to help bond fixed appliances and attachments to the tooth's enamel surface. They are used at bond-up appointments or at appointments where the orthodontic attachment has debonded away from the tooth.

Adhesives are used on many orthodontic attachments to allow for placement on a tooth. The following orthodontic attachments use an adhesive:

- Brackets, which need adhesive for placement.
- Auxiliaries such as buttons, eyelets.
- Molar bands, which need an adhesive for placement.
- Appliances: transpalatal arch (TPA), rapid maxillary expansion (RME), quadhelix, TPA with Nance.
- Archwires: adhesive used for ends of wire or for rough or sharp wire that is irritating the patient's cheek or tongue.
- Attachments on the tooth surface, such as bite turbos, bite blocks, composite buttons for elastic wear, and attachments for Invisalign treatment.

Having a fixed appliance that is bonded to the teeth allows treatment to be constant due to forces being applied 24 hours a day. Because it cannot be removed there is no worry about poor patient compliance and not achieving any tooth movement.

There are many different types of adhesives, which fall into two groups:

- Composites
- Cements.

41.2.1 Composites

A composite is a resin with filler particles that are approximately 1 μm in size. It is used to bond an orthodontic attachment to a tooth.

When bonding there is a physical adhesion between the tooth and the resin (micro-mechanical zip) and a chemical adhesion between the resin and the composite.

The composite is spread evenly onto the bonded attachment prior to placement on the tooth's enamel surface.

There are many different types of composites that can be used in orthodontics:
Light cure, for example Transbond™ (3M, St Paul, MN, USA):

- These composites have activators integrated within the solution and are activated when in contact with light.
  - Composite will still set on light cure and general light if left.

- Extended working time needed.
- 450 nm light required.
- Self-cure, for example glass ionomer cement (GIC):
  - Has two bases that are mixed together, one being the activator and one being the resin with the enzymes integrated.
  - Activator starts a chemical reaction.
  - Done on a timed system.
  - Composite sets itself.
- Dual cure, for example Grengloo™ and Blugloo™ (Ormco, Glendora, CA, USA):
  - Combines both chemical and light cure polymerization.
  - Composite is partially set by light and partially by a slower chemical reaction.
  - Initial set achieved by light curing.
  - Has a light tack set texture.
  - Has a four-minute chemical cure.
- Two paste.
- Two paste, two resin.
- Single paste and resin.
- Single paste and light.

41.2.2 Cements

The following cements can be used in orthodontics for cementing bands:

- GIC, for example Fugi LC® (GC Corporation, Tokyo, Japan) and Intact (Orthocare, Saltaire, UK):
  - Sets itself – no light cure.
  - Fluoride releasing.
  - Can reduce decalcification and decay.
  - Mixed with water to set.
  - Used for:
    - ○ Bonding brackets.
    - ○ Cementing bands.
    - ○ Bite blocks.
    - ○ Bite turbos.
    - ○ Seal under clip-on fixed functional (COFF) appliance.
  - No need for etch prior to placement.
  - Advantages:
    - ○ No etch required.
    - ○ Sets with water.
    - ○ Capsules mix in 10 seconds.
    - ○ Easier to debond than Transbond.
    - ○ Fluoride reduces decalcification and decay.
  - Disadvantages:
    - ○ Skin irritant.
    - ○ Expensive.
    - ○ Not such good bond strength.
  - GIC is the most popular cement for cementing bands because it has:
    - ○ Fluoride-releasing component.
    - ○ Affinity (natural attraction) to stainless steel and enamel.
    - ○ Use for retaining banded attachments.

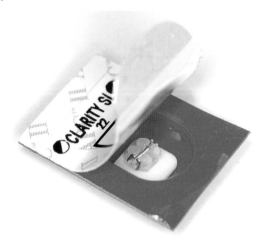

Figure 41.5 Adhesive pre-coated (APC) bracket.

- Zinc phosphate may be preferred in cementation of bands due to:
  - Relatively high compressive strength.
  - Convenient setting time.
  - Easy removal of excess cement.
- Band-Lok® (Reliance Orthodontic Products, Itasca, IL, USA).
- Poly-F® Plus (Dentsply Sirona, York, PA, USA).

41.2.3 Adhesive Pre-coated (APC) Brackets

APC brackets (Figure 41.5) come packaged with a pre-coated light cure composite already on them. Each bracket comes individually packaged.

41.3 Bonding onto Fillings, Crowns, and Veneers

41.3.1 Amalgam Fillings and Crowns

Bonding an orthodontic attachment to an amalgam filling or crown does not achieve a strong bond as opposed to bonding to a normal sound tooth. The amalgam filling/crown has to be etched as normal, however primer is needed to allow a good mechanical bond. Metal primer is then rubbed onto the tooth with a cotton pellet. Following placement of the primer, the orthodontic attachment is then placed on the tooth and light cured.

41.3.2 Porcelain Fillings/Crowns

- The tooth is etched with hydrofluoric acid 9.3%.
- Porcelain primer can be used on the tooth after etching.
- Primer is rubbed onto the tooth.
- A bracket is then placed onto the tooth and light cured.

42

Archwire Ligation

42.1 Definition of Archwire Ligation

Archwire ligation is the procedure of securing the archwire to the bracket slot.

42.2 Properties of an Ideal Ligation System

- Secure and robust.
- Ensures full archwire engagement.
- Low friction.
- Quick and easy to use.
- Permits high friction when required.
- Assists in good oral hygiene.
- Comfortable for the patient.

42.3 Methods of Ligation

The three main methods of ligation are:

1) Stainless-steel ligatures.
2) Elastomeric modules.
3) Self-ligating brackets (see Chapter 28).

42.3.1 Stainless-Steel Ligatures

Stainless-steel ligatures are used for:

- Conventional ligation.
- Rotation ties.
- Continuous ties.
- Lacebacks.
- Underties.
- Elastic wear – Kobayashi hooks.

Textbook for Orthodontic Therapists, First Edition. Ceri Davies.
© 2020 John Wiley & Sons Ltd. Published 2020 by John Wiley & Sons Ltd.

Advantages:

- Secure and robust.
- Enable full, partial, and distant ligation.
- Lower friction than elastomeric modules.

Disadvantages:

- Ends can cause trauma to soft tissues.
- Potential impediment to good oral hygiene.
- Time consuming.
- Can scratch ceramic brackets.

42.3.2 Elastomeric Modules

Elastomeric modules are another form of ligation used on conventional systems. They can be tied as a standard tie or as a figure of 8. Tying the module into a figure of 8 provides more force.
Advantages:

- Quick to use.
- Cheap.
- Comfortable for the patient.

Disadvantages:

- High friction.
- Less secure.
- Potential impediment to good oral hygiene.
- Force and therefore tooth control decay with time.
- Failure to provide full engagement of archwire.

43

Risks and Benefits of Orthodontic Treatment

43.1 Risks of Orthodontic Treatment

Risks of orthodontic treatment are categorised into three groups:

- Extra-oral risks
- Intra-oral risks
- General risks.

43.1.1 Extra-oral Risks

- Flattening of the facial profile: extractions can result in flattening of the facial profile, especially in patients with a concave profile, as this can lead the patient to look even more concave.
- Temporomandibular joint (TMJ) dysfunction, although this has not been proven.
- Ocular injuries: blindness can occur as an injury from the facebow.
- Allergies from facebow: nickel allergy can occur.

43.1.2 Intra-oral Risks

- Decalcification: can occur from poor oral hygiene (OH) and poor diet.
- Enamel fracture during debonding: incisor fracture can also occur from debonding of ceramic brackets.
- Root resorption: this can occur from excessive forces undermining resorption. Shortening of the roots occurs in all orthodontic patients (approx. 1–2 mm during fixed appliances). Other causes of root resorption are:
  - Blunt roots
  - Pipette short roots
  - Previous trauma
  - Nail biting
  - Prolonged treatment
  - Intrusion
  - Large movements

Textbook for Orthodontic Therapists, First Edition. Ceri Davies.
© 2020 John Wiley & Sons Ltd. Published 2020 by John Wiley & Sons Ltd.

- Torque
- Intermaxillary elastics.

- Gingivitis/gingival hyperplasia due to poor OH during treatment. Inflamed gums can occur from tooth movement.
- Uncontrolled pre-existing periodontitis: appliances can make this more critical.
- Periodontal attachment loss due to poor OH.
- Loss of vitality can occur to teeth that have suffered previous trauma.
- Ulcerations: trauma on mucosa from appliances due to rubbing, excess wire, etc.

43.1.3   General Risks

- Pain: tenderness to teeth due to tooth movement and irritation of the mucosa.
- Poor patient satisfaction: lack of communication between staff and patients.
- Patients' expectations: these may be too high.
- Poor communication between staff and patients.
- Poor compliance: patient not doing what they are advised.
- Poor retention: lack of communication and instructions not taken on board.
- Radiation: exposure to radiation from radiographs.
- No treatment option: risks if patient chooses no treatment option need to be explained.

43.2   Benefits of Orthodontic Treatment

Benefits of orthodontic treatment are categorised into three groups:

- Psychological benefits
- Dental health benefits
- Functional benefits.

43.2.1   Psychological Benefits

- Improved self-esteem.
- Improved confidence.
- Improved social interaction.
- Stopping bullying at school, for example due to an increased overjet.

43.2.2   Dental Health Benefits

- Reduced risk of trauma. For example, an increased overjet is less lightly to suffer trauma if reduced. Deepbites can result in tooth wear and periodontal destruction and an edge-to-edge bite can result in wear of the enamel.
- Improved OH because of relieved crowding.
- Improved periodontal health.
- Mastication: helps with incision and chewing of food.
- Stopping habits: digit sucking habit and adaptive tongue thrust.

- Aesthetics: achieving a more aesthetically pleasing smile.
- Reduces risk of root resorption of adjacent teeth from impacted teeth.
- Hypodontia: closed spaces or open spaces for prosthetics such as implants or bridges.

43.2.3 Functional Benefits

- Improvement to speech.
- Improvement to TMJ, although that is not proven.
- Mastication: help with incision and chewing of food.

44

Oral Hygiene

Oral hygiene (OH) is the practice of keeping the mouth and teeth clean to prevent dental problems, most commonly dental cavities, gingivitis, and bad breath (halitosis).

44.1   Oral Hygiene: Pre-treatment

OH must be of a good standard before orthodontic treatment can be commenced. Any patient who presents with bad OH at the initial assessment cannot proceed to treatment without improving this first. Patients must be given OH instructions and reviewed until they can maintain a good standard of OH.

The following steps must be considered for patients who present with bad OH:

- Delay treatment until OH has improved.
- Give instructions on improving OH and make patient aware of the importance of good OH.
- Review patient until good OH is being maintained.
- Show patient photos damaged teeth from poor OH with orthodontic treatment such as decalcification.
- Take pre-treatment photos of patient's OH condition and review and compare these with OH on review appointments.
- Look at gingival health compare how good OH is there.

44.2   Clinical Features for Good and Bad Oral Hygiene

Good OH (Figures 44.1 and 44.2):

- Healthy gums – light pink gingiva.
- No plaque build-up around teeth or brackets.
- No inflammation around the gingival margin of the gums.
- No staining.
- No food debris.
- No bleeding of the gums when brushing.

Textbook for Orthodontic Therapists, First Edition. Ceri Davies.
© 2020 John Wiley & Sons Ltd. Published 2020 by John Wiley & Sons Ltd.

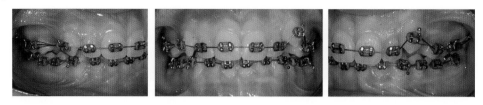

Figure 44.1 Centric and buccal views of good oral hygiene. Intra-oral photographs at the start of treatment.

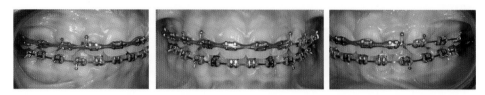

Figure 44.2 Centric and buccal views of good oral hygiene. Intra-oral photographs mid-treatment.

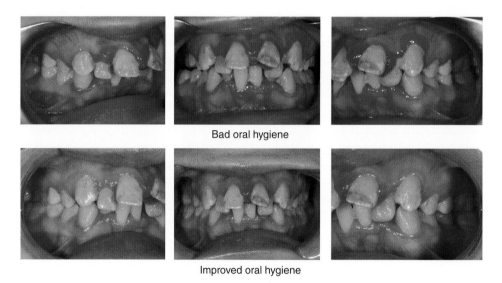

Bad oral hygiene

Improved oral hygiene

Figure 44.3 Centric and buccal views of bad and improved oral hygiene.

Bad OH (Figure 44.3):

- Unhealthy gums – swollen and red, with gingival hyperplasia.
- Inflammation on the gingival margin.
- Plaque build-up around brackets and teeth.
- Build-up of food debris.
- Staining present.
- Bleeding gums when brushing.
- Decalcification present once braces are off.

44.3 Procedure with Patients Presenting with Bad Oral Hygiene

Patients presenting with bad OH must have the correct advice and an opportunity to improve. Anyone presenting with bad OH should first have clinical photographs taken. The photographs will help show the patient the areas they are missing and identify the areas or area that needs improvement. After giving the patient instructions, it is good to show the patient the improvement in OH, if any has been made, at the following visit by use of the photographs.

The following instructions should be given to the patient:

- Two minutes spent brushing with fluoride toothpaste every morning and evening – three seconds on each tooth:
  - Manual toothbrush – circular motions on each tooth.
  - Electric toothbrush – hold toothbrush on each tooth.
  - Do not rinse with water but leave toothpaste in the mouth, which allows for fluoride to soak into the teeth.
- Flossing or tepee brushes: morning and evening floss between the teeth and high up on the gum margin. If there is bleeding carry on, do not do less.
- Fluoride mouthwash: use twice during the day, once late morning and again late afternoon. This allows for fluoride intake during the day.
- Use a plaque-disclosing tablet.

Show the patients the instructions for tooth cleaning on typodonts. Also show them pictures of damaged teeth and decalcification. If there is no change on review appointments, delay treatment further or do not start it.

44.4 Procedure with Patients Who Have Improvement in Oral Hygiene

Once patients have improved their OH, the following procedure must be carried out:

- Agree to start treatment.
- Advise patient that the improved OH must carry on throughout treatment and the rest of their lives if they want healthy teeth.
- Get consent:
  - Stress the importance of good OH.
  - Advise that chocolates, sweets, and fizzy drinks should be eaten/drunk rarely, and if they are, at mealtimes only. Suggest to parents that they do not buy fizzy drinks for their children.
- Tell the patient that braces will be removed if their subsequent OH is poor.

44.5 Oral Hygiene Advice Given at the Fit Appointment

- Give instructions on maintenance of cleaning. Show cleaning on typodont.
- Show a DVD illustrating the advice.
- Give the patient a toothbrush kit.

- Give advice about potential issues with braces:
  - Toothache.
  - Remove for sports if appliance is removable.
  - Fixed – use mouthguard.
  - Wax – use for trauma.
  - Trauma to soft tissues – ulcers.
  - Pain/tenderness – pain relief tablets.

44.6   Preventing Decalcification

- Strongly advise the patient that they have to improve their OH and stress its importance.
- Warn the patient that if their OH is not better by the next visit, the braces will be removed and treatment will be stopped.
- If a child, send a letter to the parent(s) warning them about the bad OH.
- Take wire out.
- Take brace off completely.

44.7   Oral Hygiene Instructions for Appliances

44.7.1   Removable Appliance

- Electric toothbrush/manual toothbrush:
  - Spend two minutes cleaning your teeth every morning and evening.
  - If you use an electric toothbrush, hold it on each tooth for three seconds.
  - If you use a manual toothbrush, do circular motions on each tooth for three seconds.
- Floss/tepee brushes:
  - Floss can be used to clean between the teeth and gum margin.
  - Tepee brushes can also do the same job in the appropriate sizes.
- Mouthwash:
  - Use mouthwash twice a day, ideally late morning and late afternoon, for a regular fluoride intake.
- Cleaning of the appliance:
  - Clean the appliance when cleaning your teeth morning and evening.
  - Clean the appliance after eating to remove any food debris caught within the brace.
  - Use toothbrush and toothpaste to clean the appliance or use Retainer Brite, a tablet that dissolves in warm water in which the appliance can be put to clean and sterilise it.

44.7.2   Functional Appliance

- Electric toothbrush/manual toothbrush:
  - Spend two minutes cleaning your teeth every morning and evening.
  - If you use an electric toothbrush, hold it on each tooth for three seconds.
  - If you use a manual toothbrush, do circular motions on each tooth for three seconds.
- Floss/tepee brushes:
  - Floss can be used to clean between the teeth and gum margin
  - Tepee brushes can also do the same job in the appropriate sizes.

- Mouthwash:
  - Use mouthwash twice a day, ideally late morning and late afternoon, for a regular fluoride intake.
- Cleaning of the appliance:
  - Clean the appliance when cleaning your teeth morning and evening.
  - Clean the appliance after eating to remove any food debris caught within the brace.
  - Use toothbrush and toothpaste to clean the appliance or use Retainer Brite, a tablet that dissolves in warm water in which the appliance can be put to clean and sterilise it.

44.7.3 Fixed Appliance

- Avoid any bright or richly coloured foods for 48 hours after your fixed brace is fitted, as they may stain your teeth permanently.
  - Foods to avoid: ketchup, soup, brown sauce, mustard, baked beans, curries, etc.
  - Foods/drinks you can have: water, milk, lemonade, plain pasta, white cheese, potatoes, fish, chips, any bland-coloured foods.
- Orthodontic brush/conventional brush:
  - Spend four minutes every morning and evening cleaning your teeth and brace.
  - Spend two minutes on your teeth, doing circular motions on each tooth for three seconds.
  - Spend two minutes on your brace, cleaning around your brace, under the archwires, and around the brackets and bands.
- Interspace brush:
  - Use this brush to clean underneath each archwire between the brackets to remove any plaque or food debris.
- Tepee brushes:
  - Use these brushes to clean around each side of the bracket to remove any plaque build-up and food debris. Doing this will prevent staining around the brackets, which can lead to decalcification.
  - If of an appropriate size, these brushes can be used between the teeth as an alternative to floss.
- Floss:
  - Floss can be used to clean around the brackets as an alternative to tepee brushes.
  - Floss can also be used to feed underneath the archwire and between the teeth to clean the contact points and gum margin.
- Mouthwash:
  - Fluoride mouthwash should not be used for the first three days as it could permanently stain your teeth.
  - After that, use mouthwash twice a day, ideally late morning and late afternoon, for a fluoride intake throughout the day.
- Disclosing tablets:
  - Disclosing tablets should not be used for the first three days as they could permanently stain your teeth.
  - After that, use these tablets occasionally to make sure you are cleaning properly.
  - Chew the tablet for about a minute after cleaning and then spit it out. Any areas of dark purple and light purple on your teeth are built-up areas of plaque that you have missed when cleaning.
- Diet:
  - Avoid foods which can cause breakages or other damage: hard/sticky foods and fizzy drinks, including crusty bread, toffees, hard nuts, bubblegum/chewing gum, pizza crusts.

45

Decalcification

Decalcification is where teeth lose calcium. When calcium is lost, demineralisation of the enamel happens, which can be due to acid erosion. Decalcification is also an early stage of tooth decay.

Decalcification can appear differently: in mild cases it can appear as white lesions on the teeth, whereas in severe cases it will appear as brown lesions that lead to caries. Figure 45.1 is a mild case of decalcification where the white lesions can be seen on the teeth.

45.1 Causes of Decalcification

There are three main factors that cause decalcification:

- *Plaque build-up due to poor oral hygiene (OH):* bacteria found in dental plaque will convert carbohydrates and sugars into acids.
- *Diet:* bacteria found in plaque will feed off sugars in patients who have a high sugar intake in their diet; the bacteria will convert into acid, causing demineralization of the enamel.
- *Fixed appliances:* poor OH can result in plaque accumulating around brackets and under the archwires due to the patient not removing it efficiently. Patients who have poor OH are more prone to decalcification.

45.2 Occurrence of Decalcification

In orthodontics, 80–85% of patients experience decalcification. Patients who do not brush their teeth properly are more prone to decalcification. Those who present with poor OH must be informed of the risk of damage to their teeth they are doing. Photographs of different cases of decalcification should be available to show patients what can happen to their teeth if they do not improve their OH.

Any patient presenting with bad OH should be made aware of it and given the chance to improve, and the clinician should give them instructions on how to do so. It may even be a good approach to go through cleaning techniques at the patient's appointment using the toothbrush, tepee brushes, floss, and interspace brush they get in their orthodontic cleaning kits. Plaque disclosing tablets are a good tool to use in the dental chair, as they can show the patient the areas they may be missing. Clinical photographs of the patient's bad OH should be taken, as they can be used four weeks later alongside new photographs at their follow-up appointment, and reviewed with the patient to demonstrate any improvement.

Textbook for Orthodontic Therapists, First Edition. Ceri Davies.
© 2020 John Wiley & Sons Ltd. Published 2020 by John Wiley & Sons Ltd.

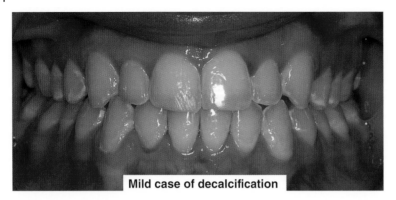

Figure 45.1 Mild case of decalcification.

Following the first review, if the patient's OH is still not good enough the archwires should be removed, and the patient be given another four weeks to improve. If there is still no improvement, consideration must be given to discontinuing treatment.

45.3 Preventing Decalcification

There are four main ways in which decalcification can be prevented, by the patient themselves and by the clinician.

- *Good OH:*
  - It is important to ensure that the patient has been given good OH instructions by the clinician.
  - All patients must ensure that they are keeping up with their OH at all times throughout treatment.
- *Dietary advice:*
  - Patient must be aware that they will need to limit their sugar intake. If they are to have any sugary foods, these must be eaten at meal times. The reason is that when we eat there is a drop in the pH level and the acidity level decreases from 6 to 1. A constant drop in the pH level between meals increases the risk of demineralization of the enamel, potentially leading to caries. A pH below 5.5 results in an acid attack to the teeth. A neutral pH value is 7.
- *Use of fluoride toothpaste/mouthwash*:
  - All patients must be using a fluoride toothpaste and mouthwash, to ensure that they are getting their daily intake of fluoride.
- *Auxiliaries:*
  - To help prevent poor OH, clinicians should avoid using elastomeric modules, as they attract plaque. Consideration should be given to using stainless-steel quick ligatures or fluoride-releasing modules.

45.4 Treating Decalcification

Decalcification can be treated via a procedure called enameloplasty, which removes some of the tooth surface by using 18% hydrofluoric acid mixed in pumice. By doing this the appearance of the decalcification is improved. If this is considered, it is usually done three months after lesions are stabilised.

46

Fluorosis

Fluorosis is a disturbance in the development of the enamel that is caused by excessive consumption of fluoride during the tooth development stage. Fluorosis is also known as mottling of the tooth enamel.

Fluorosis can appear differently: in milder cases it will appear as tiny white streaks/specks or spots within the enamel, whereas severe cases will present as discoloration or brown markings/stains within the enamel. Figure 46.1 is a mild case of fluorosis located on the teeth.

46.1 How Can Fluorosis Occur?

From the age of 1–4 years, children are at risk of fluorosis if they consume an excessive amount of fluoride. Fluoride is not just found in the toothpaste and mouthwash that we use daily to clean our teeth, but can also be found in bottled water, foods we eat, and even water in public areas. It is important that during this stage all children are supervised when cleaning their teeth to ensure they do not swallow any of the toothpaste with its fluoride content. Children are no longer at risk of fluorosis after the age of 8 years, once the teeth have erupted into the oral cavity, as by this point the crown of the tooth is fully developed.

46.2 Products That Can Cause Fluorosis

The following products can contain fluoride and cause fluorosis:

- Fluoride mouthwash
- Fluoride toothpaste
- Bottled water that is not tested for its fluoride content
- Foods
- Public water supply – fluoridation varies between areas.

Textbook for Orthodontic Therapists, First Edition. Ceri Davies.
© 2020 John Wiley & Sons Ltd. Published 2020 by John Wiley & Sons Ltd.

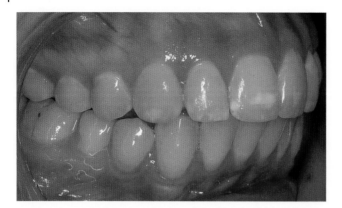

Figure 46.1 Right buccal view of fluorosis.

46.3 Treating Fluorosis

Doing the following can treat fluorosis cosmetically:

- Bleaching
- Micro-abrasion
- Composite restorations
- Porcelain veneers.

46.4 Preventing Fluorosis

Fluorosis can be prevented in the following ways:

- Children under 8 years old should have toothbrushing supervised by an adult to prevent ingestion of the toothpaste.
- Use a minimum amount of toothpaste – the size of a small pea – and use it twice a day only.
- Ensure that toothpaste is spat out and not swallowed.

47

Fluoride

Fluoride is a salt which can be added to water supplies or toothpaste to help reduce tooth decay. It helps to strengthen teeth, making them less prone to an acid attack and damage by dental caries.

47.1 Effects of Fluoride

Fluoride affects the teeth by:

- Increasing mineralisation.
- Reducing demineralisation.
- Decreasing acid production in plaque.
- Reducing the amount of bacteria in the mouth.

47.2 Toothpaste Ingredients

Toothpaste contains the following ingredients:

- *Sodium fluoride*: helps to strengthen enamel and remineralise the tooth surface.
- *Abrasives*: remove debris and residual surface stains.

47.3 Dental Products

Different amounts of fluoride are found within the dental products we use today:

- Toothpaste: 1450 ppm
- Mouthwash (Fluorigard Daily, Colgate-Palmolive, Guildford, UK): 0.05%–22 ppm
- Duraphat® (Colgate-Palmolive; as used by dentists): 22 600 ppm
- Prescribed Duraphat: 5000 ppm.

Textbook for Orthodontic Therapists, First Edition. Ceri Davies.
© 2020 John Wiley & Sons Ltd. Published 2020 by John Wiley & Sons Ltd.

47.4   Fluoride Application

Fluoride can be applied topically, that is directly into the enamel structure. The following products contain topical fluoride, which is useful in orthodontics:

- Toothpaste
- Mouthwash
- Fluoride gels/varnish
- Fluoride-releasing cements such as glass ionomer
- Fluoride-releasing elastomeric modules.

Fluoride can also be applied systemically, via food and drink products, such as drinking water in some areas. Foods such as rice, pasta and vegetables can contain fluoride if they are boiled in fluoridated water.

47.5   Risks of Fluoride

Excessive consumption of fluoride can have an effect on the teeth. If too much fluoride is swallowed at around the age of 1–4 years old, there is a risk of staining/mottling and fluorosis (see Chapter 46).

After the age of 8 children are no longer at risk, although until the teeth fully erupt into the oral cavity there is still a small possibility of fluorosis. Once they have erupted there is no longer a risk due to the crown being fully developed.

47.6   Other Causes and Conditions Which Can Affect Enamel Development

There are many other factors that can have an effect on enamel development, such as:

- Infections – rubella, measles
- Amelogenesis
- Hypoparathyroidism
- Drugs
- Nutritional deficiencies
- Premature birth
- Haematological and metabolic disorders.

48

Hypoplastic Enamel

Hypoplastic enamel is a defect in the enamel surface due to fewer minerals within the enamel. This can appear brown and the tooth/teeth are more porous and more prone to bracket failures. Brackets being bonded onto a tooth that has enamel hypoplasia must have the etch left on the tooth for double the time, and even possibly etched twice. Figures 48.1 and 48.2 are clinical photographs of enamel hypoplasia.

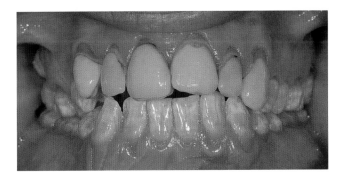

Figure 48.1   Centric view of enamel hypoplasia with veneers on the upper anterior teeth.

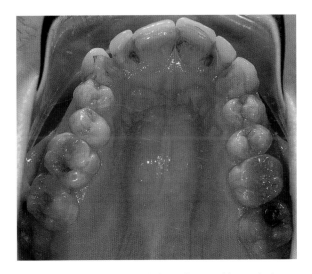

Figure 48.2   Upper occlusal view of enamel hypoplasia.

Textbook for Orthodontic Therapists, First Edition. Ceri Davies.
© 2020 John Wiley & Sons Ltd. Published 2020 by John Wiley & Sons Ltd.

48.1   Aetiology of Enamel Hypoplasia

Causes of enamel hypoplasia can include the following:

- Trauma.
- Environmental damage: disruption of ameloblast cells that make tooth enamel due to a fever, malnutrition, or hypocalcaemia whilst teeth were forming during foetal development.
- Bacterial infection.
- Slow enamel formation.
- Coeliac disease.

49

Hyperplastic Enamel

Hyperplastic enamel is a defect in the enamel of a tooth surface, because of excess minerals within the enamel. It can appear white and creamy and the tooth/teeth are similar to a patient who has enamel hypoplasia, resulting in the teeth being more porous and more prone to bracket failures. Leaving the etch on the tooth for double the time and etching twice are both to be considered. Figure 49.1 is a clinical photograph of enamel hyperplasia.

49.1 Aetiology of Enamel Hyperplasia

The causes of enamel hyperplasia are the same as those of enamel hypoplastia:

- Trauma.
- Environmental damage: disruption of ameloblast cells that make tooth enamel due to a fever, malnutrition, or hypocalcaemia while teeth were forming during foetal development.
- Bacterial infection.
- Slow enamel formation.
- Coeliac disease.

Both enamel hypoplasia and enamel hyperplasia are classified under enamel hypoplasia.

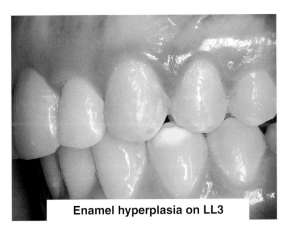

Enamel hyperplasia on LL3

Figure 49.1   Enamel hyperplasia on LL3.

Textbook for Orthodontic Therapists, First Edition. Ceri Davies.
© 2020 John Wiley & Sons Ltd. Published 2020 by John Wiley & Sons Ltd.

50

General Dental Council (GDC)

The General Dental Council (GDC) is the regulating body in the UK of all dental professionals, including specialists, dentists, hygienists, dental therapists, orthodontic therapists, dental technicians, clinical dental technicians, and nurses. Its main purpose is to protect the patient's safety and maintain public confidence in dental services. Each qualified dental care professional (DCP) has to be registered with the GDC and has to obey the standards it sets out.

Having all DCPs registered helps the GDC ensure that every professional is of a very good standard to work on patients, after gaining the appropriate education and qualifications they need to practice in the UK. This also ensures that every dental professional is fit to practice and that anyone who falls short of the standards will undergo further investigation. The GDC protects patients as well as promoting confidence within the dental profession, and is at the forefront of health-care regulations.

50.1   Roles of the GDC

The GDC has the following roles:

- Registering DCPs:
  - All dental professionals, once qualified, must be registered with the GDC to be able to practise in the UK.
  - Any person who is found practising without being registered will be prosecuted through the courts by the GDC. This may involve a prison sentence or a heavy fine, depending on the case.
- Setting standards of education:
  - Every dental professional must obey the standards that are set out by the GDC.
  - These include standards of education.
  - Any professional who does not undergo education that is verified by the GDC will be unable to gain entry to the register.
- Setting standards of dental practice and conduct:
  - Every dental professional must obey the standards of dental practice and conduct, which are represented by the nine GDC principles that must be followed (discussed in the next section).
  - Any professional who does not follow these principles will be investigated further by the Fitness to Practice panel.

Textbook for Orthodontic Therapists, First Edition. Ceri Davies.
© 2020 John Wiley & Sons Ltd. Published 2020 by John Wiley & Sons Ltd.

- Ensuring DCPs are keeping up to date by continuing professional development (CPD):
  - All DCPs are required to carry out CPD.
  - Every professional has a different number of hours they require to undertake within a five-year cycle.
  - Dentists require 150 hours, DCPs 75 hours, nurses 50 hours.
- Helping patients with complaints:
  - Any complaints made against a dental professional can involve the GDC.
  - Patients can get in contact with the GDC about any professional who is deemed to be unfit to practice. This will then require further investigation by the GDC.
  - Depending on how serious the compliant is, it can result in the professional being sued and possibly struck off or suspended for a certain amount of time.
- Working to strengthen patient protection:
  - The GDC works to strengthen patient protection by keeping standards of education, dental practice, and conduct up to date and ensuring all dental professionals are adhering to these.
  - The GDC also has the right to investigate any professional who fails to follow its standards.

50.2 GDC Principles

The GDC principles are standards that are set out by the GDC that all dental professionals have to follow. These prescribe standards of dental practice and conduct. Originally there were only six principles, but in 2013 they changed to nine and all DCPs registered with the GDC were notified by being issued with a standards booklet. This contains all the standards that all registrants have to adhere to, with guidance for each standard. The guidance helps dental professionals meet the standards by knowing what is expected of them.

The principles include standards of ethics, performance, and conduct and are all equally important and not in any order of priority. They represent what every dental professional must do, and anyone who does not carry out or meet these standards can be removed from the register and will not be able to work within the profession any more. The GDC has the authority to admonish, suspend, or remove from the register any dental professional who is found to have any impaired fitness to practice.

The nine GDC principles are:

1) Put patients' interests first.
2) Communicate effectively with patients.
3) Obtain valid consent.
4) Maintain and protect patients' information.
5) Have a clear and effective complaints procedure.
6) Work with colleagues in a way that is in patients' best interest.
7) Maintain, develop and work within your professional knowledge and skills.
8) Raise concerns if patients are at risk.
9) Make sure your personal behaviour maintains patients' confidence in you and the dental profession. (https://standards.gdc-uk.org)

Detailed descriptions of the patient's expectations and what each principle requires can be found in more detail in the standards booklet for the dental team.

50.3 Continuing Professional Development

CPD is a requirement that is to be met by all dental professionals registered with the GDC. This was first introduced in 2008 and has been made a legal requirement that everyone has to carry out to keep and maintain their registration. CPD was introduced to ensure that all professionals are keeping up to date with their knowledge and skills to benefit patients.

Over a five-year cycle, dentists used to have to carry out 250 hours of CPD, while other dental professionals had a requirement for 150 hours, split into verifiable and non-verifiable development. Verifiable CPD involves documentary evidence of the CPD undertaken, which can be in the form of a certificate with the DCP's name on, their GDC number, the title of the CPD completed, and how many hours it is worth. Details of all verifiable CPD had to be kept for proven evidence of meeting the GDC requirements. Non-verifiable CPD does not require any evidence and is done so that the DCP can continue development in their profession, maintaining patient confidence. For dentists 75 verifiable hours were required, with 175 being non-verifiable; for the remaining DCPs it was 50 verifiable hours and 100 non-verifiable.

In August 2018 the GDC changed the way CPD was done by all registrants. Non-verifiable CPD was removed and only verifiable ECPD (enhanced continuing professional development) is now required. Changing this and removing the non-verifiable element increased the verifiable hours over the five-year cycle. Dentists are now required to do 150 hours, DCPs 75 hours, and nurses 50 hours within the five years. A few other changes were also brought in. First, a professional development plan (PDP) is expected, with each registrant required to fill one out each year to plan the topics of the CPD they are going to do for that year. Verifiable ECPD also requires documentary evidence such as certificates and reflective learning on the subject/course. Reflective learning allows the DCP to reflect on the topic of the ECPD they have done, asking themselves what they have learnt, how they will apply this to their daily duties, and how they are going to maintain this knowledge. After filling out the reflective learning record, the registrant is required to fill out a CPD Activity Log. This is documentary evidence that ties in with the PDP. The importance of the CPD Activity Log is that it provides written evidence of all the ECPD each registrant has undertaken and is a requirement for any ECPD to be considered verifiable. Figure 50.1 is an example of what a CPD Activity Log should look like and what information is needed for each section.

The CPD Activity Log should be kept with all the certificates from all CPD completed. It can either be saved electronically or printed out and kept in a folder along with all the original certificates. It does not matter how it is saved as long as it is updated after completion of any CPD and is easily accessible if the GDC requests it.

Registrants cannot complete just any ECPD they want through the five-year cycle. The GDC sets topics for essential CPD and recommended CPD. *Essential* CPD is CPD that every DCP has to complete within the five-year cycle, with a required number of hours. Anyone who does not complete this can risk losing their registration. *Recommended* CPD covers topics that the GDC only advises should be done: these subjects are not a requirement, but they are highly recommended.

The essential CPD that is required by the GDC is:

- Medical emergencies – ten hours in every five-year cycle.
- Disinfection and decontamination – five hours in every five-year cycle.
- Radiographs and radiation – five hours in every five-year cycle.

Name: GDC Number: Cycle Period:

Date	Hours completed	Evidence of verifiable CPD? (e.g. certificate)	Title, provider and content of CPD activity	Development outcome(s)	How did this activity benefit my daily work?
The dates you completed the CPD	*The amount of verifiable hours confirmed by the certificate for the CPD completed*	*What type of evidence do you have to provide proof that the CPD was completed?*	*This section should contain the title of the CPD, who provided it and what was covered in the CPD activity*	*A, B, C, D* *The CPD must indicate the development outcomes of the CPD*	*This section is where you reflect back on the CPD you have completed. When reflecting you should consider the following:* *What was learnt from the CPD you completed, was it helpful or relevant to your daily work and patients?* *Was there any changes/updates towards your daily work, if so what are they and how did you make the changes?* *If there were no changes/updates what did the CPD confirm for you that you may already know or be doing?* *What is the benefit of you completing this CPD and how does it improve your daily work and benefit your patients?*

Figure 50.1 CPD Activity Log.

The recommended CPD that the GDC advises is:

- Legal and ethical issues.
- Complaints handling.
- Oral cancers – early detection.
- Safeguarding children and young people.
- Safeguarding vulnerable adults.

Every DCP registered with the GDC has an eGDC account. This is accessed online and allows registrants to log in and declare their CPD, manage their registration online, pay the associated registration fees, and complete their annual renewal process. The CPD section is where all registrants can log their CPD. On this page each year in their cycle is divided into sections with a drop-down menu where hours can be logged, only as whole numbers. CPD that is logged must have been undertaken within that year and any previous CPD that was not logged cannot be added to a year in which it was not completed. When declaring the CPD each registrant must confirm the following:

- I have read and understand the CPD requirements.
- The hours recorded in this statement have been undertaken during this CPD year.
- That I have kept a CPD record (including a personal development plan).
- The CPD undertaken (where applicable) was relevant to my field of practice.
- The information contained in this statement is full and accurate.

Each registrant must confirm that this is true every time they update their CPD. At the end of every dental professional's five-year cycle, all CPD has to have been submitted on their eGDC. The GDC will select at random a number of registrants whose cycle has finished and require them to provide documentary evidence of all the CPD they have completed within that five-year cycle. It is impossible to know if you will be chosen, so keeping up to date with all CPD is a must. Anyone who fails to provide evidence to the GDC will be further investigated, resulting in a risk of losing their registration.

50.4   GDC Register

All dental professionals must be listed on the GDC register. When any dental professional qualifies, they must inform the GDC by filling out the appropriate paperwork. The GDC must also be notified of any DCP who gains a further qualification, such as a registered dental nurse who may have qualified as an orthodontic therapist, as their registration will need to be updated.

There are three separate registers for the following:

- Dentists
- DCPs
- Specialists.

It is illegal to work as a DCP in the UK without being registered with the GDC. Any DCP found to be practising in the UK without being registered will be seen as unfit to practise and will be further investigated, resulting in them being sued and never being able to practise again in the UK.

When placed on the register, every registrant is supplied with a GDC number and a certificate. Every registrant has to pay a fee each year, as GDC registration only lasts for one year. This fee can be paid in different ways, either by setting up a direct debit, a one-off payment made each year, or via the eGDC account. Any registrant who misses a payment is automatically removed from the register and is immediately unable to work.

Furthermore, every registrant must make sure they have their own indemnity insurance. This is not supplied by the GDC and is available via companies such as Dental Protection or the Medical Protection Society (MPS). Under no circumstances should any DCP be working without indemnity insurance. Every year as well as paying the annual fee every DCP has to declare they have indemnity insurance when renewing via the eGDC account, and any false declaration would result in the DCP being struck off of the register and possibly result in them no longer being able to work in the profession again.

50.5   Professional Conduct Committee

The Professional Conduct Committee (PCC) is a statutory committee of the GDC. It investigates any allegation made against a dental professional and decides whether this represents unacceptable behaviour, which can result in withdrawing the registrant's ability to work within the profession. Members of the committee are drawn from the Fitness to Practice panel and are either lay members or dental professionals.

There are 10 reasons why a DCP may be referred to the GDC/PCC for further investigation:

1) Poor treatment.
2) Fraud, unjustified claims, wrong charging.
3) Prescribing issues.
4) Conscious sedation issues.
5) No indemnity insurance.
6) Poor practice management.
7) Basis of treatment (NHS/private).
8) Cross-infection control issues.
9) Failure to obtain valid consent/explain treatment.
10) Failure to carry out work under direction of dentist/orthodontist.

After an allegation has been made, the PCC has to:

- Decide whether the registrant's fitness to practice is impaired. If it is not, it will cease the case.
- In cases where it has been impaired, issue a reprimand.
- Or set conditions the registrant has to follow for up to 36 months followed by a review, which can take effect immediately.
- Or suspend the registrant for up to 12 months with or without a review, which can take effect immediately.
- Or completely erase the registrant from the register.

The PCC thus has various options for dealing with a DCP who has been found guilty of unacceptable behaviour:

- *Reprimand*: a statement of disapproval from the committee. The registrant is still considered fit to practice, with no restrictions or actions needed to be taken.
- *Conditions*: the committee issues restrictions on the registrant for a set amount of time.
- *Suspension*: the committee can suspend the registration for a set amount of time, which means the registrant cannot work within that time.
- *Erasure*: the registrant is completely erased from the register and can no longer work in the profession in the UK. This is the most serious outcome.

Registrants who find themselves up against the PCC do have the right to appeal against its findings. Hearings are held at the CCT Venues-Smithfield conference centre in London, or on some occasions at the GDC in Wimpole Street, London.

The police have the authority to inform the GDC of any cautions or convictions a dental professional has been given. When the GDC is notified of this, the PCC will investigate further to decide whether this is a fitness to practice issue.

50.6 Scope of Practice

The orthodontic therapist's scope of practice can be found on the GDC website. All therapists must ensure they know their scope of practice inside out. Lack of awareness can result in causing harm to the patient and performing procedures they should not be doing. Any therapist found not to know their scope of practice is considered unfit to practice, which can have the consequence of referral to the GDC.

The orthodontic therapist's scope of practice involves the following areas.

50.6.1 What Orthodontic Therapists Can Do

Orthodontic therapists are allowed to do the following:

- *Identify, select, maintain, and use appropriate instruments*:
  - It is important that every orthodontic therapist knows the orthodontic instruments they are using and can locate which ones they need to work with for each type of orthodontic appliance. Failure to do this can result in damage to the teeth and appliances.
- *Give instructions on oral hygiene and care of appliances*:
  - Every therapist must be able to give appropriate and efficient oral hygiene instructions. Failing to do this results in neglect and is not working in the patient's best interests, resulting in the DCP not meeting the GDC standards.

- *Make referrals to other health-care professionals*:
  - Orthodontic therapists must be able to identify when they need to refer a patient to a specialist orthodontist and other health-care professionals, such as a hygienist for patients who are presenting with poor oral hygiene that needs maintaining and improving.
- *Make appliances safe in the absence of a dentist*:
  - Orthodontic therapists must be able to know the limits of being able to make orthodontic appliances safe, such as getting the patient out of discomfort by cutting a long wire or rebonding a bracket. Any appliance that is embedded in the mouth such as a transpalatal arch embedded in the palate should be referred to the orthodontist. If the orthodontist is not present on the day, the therapist should be aware they need to send the patient to the Accident and Emergency Department if they are in pain or to tell them to come back and see the orthodontist another time.
- *Take occlusal records and orthognathic facebow readings*
  - Orthodontic therapists who work in the Maxillofacial Department in a hospital can take occlusal records and orthognathic facebow readings on patients who are going to be having orthodontics followed by surgery.
- *Fit removable appliances that have been previously activated by the orthodontist*:
  - Orthodontic therapists are only allowed to adjust retentive components on a removable appliance. Any active components must be activated by the orthodontist. However, after activation the appliance can be fitted by the therapist.
- *Fit passive removable appliances*:
  - The therapist can fit passive appliances such as retainers.
- *Adjust retentive components*:
  - Only retentive components are to be adjusted by the therapist to ensure the appliance is secure in the mouth. Any active components must be adjusted by the orthodontist.
- *Prepare tooth surface for fixed appliance placement*:
  - Preparation of a tooth surface for fixed appliances involves etching, bonding, placing the attachment onto the tooth, and setting it with a light cure.
- *Placing separators, brackets, and bands*:
  - Therapists are able to place separators between contact points of teeth, cement molar bands into place, and bond brackets onto teeth.
- *Bond fixed appliances*:
  - All therapists can bond fixed appliances to the teeth following the correct procedure for preparing the tooth surface, such as etching, bond, composite placement with attachment, and light cure.
- *Insert, ligate, and remove archwires*:
  - Therapists can see patients at fixed adjustment appointments following the written prescription of the orthodontist. This involves the therapist removing the archwire, inserting a new archwire, and ligating it to the teeth by use of quick ligatures, elastomeric modules, or closing the door on a self-ligating bracket, depending on the system being used.
- *Remove fixed appliances and composites/cements – debonding*:
  - Following instructions from the orthodontist, therapists can remove fixed appliances and polish composites and cements with the use of a slow handpiece and tungsten carbide bur.
- *Fit headgear that has been previously activated by the orthodontist*:
  - Activation of the facebow must be done by the orthodontist. However, therapists are able to fit an active facebow after it has been adjusted by the orthodontist.
- *Take impressions and photographs*:
  - Impressions can be taken by the orthodontic therapist for study models, for manufacture of an orthodontic appliance that has been prescribed by the orthodontist, and for retainers at the

end of treatment. Therapists can also take photographs which are needed for records, such as initial records, mid-treatment, and final records. Any therapist who has gained qualifications in taking radiographs can also take the appropriate radiographs for the patient, but only after a prescription from the orthodontist.

- *Pour, cast, and trim models*:
  - Therapists can also pour, cast, and trim models from the impressions taken for study models and in-house retainers if there is a lab on site within the practice.

50.6.2 What Orthodontic Therapists Cannot Do

Orthodontic therapists cannot do the following:

- *Diagnose and treatment plan*:
  - No therapist is allowed to diagnose patients and plan treatment; this is for only the orthodontist to do.
- *Remove subgingival calculus*:
  - No therapist is allowed to remove subgingival calculus. If any is present the patient should be advised or referred to the hygienist for removal and maintenance.
- *Place temporary dressings*:
  - No therapist is allowed to place any temporary dressings; this must be done by the orthodontist.
- *Give local anaesthetic*:
  - No therapist is allowed to give a local anaesthetic to a patient; this is done only by the orthodontist.
- *Re-cement crowns*:
  - Any crowns that come loose during orthodontic treatment cannot be re-cemented by the therapist. Either the orthodontist does this if there is an appropriate cement in the practice, or the patient is to be referred back to their dentist to have this done.
- *Use a fast handpiece*:
  - Fast handpieces are sometimes needed during orthodontic treatment for possible interproximal reduction (IPR) or removal of a bracket that is fractured. If this is the case, only orthodontists are allowed to do this. Therapists can only use a slow handpiece to remove any cements or composites and a straight handpiece to smooth acrylic on a removable appliance.
- *Do IPR*:
  - IPR is sometimes needed on patients to create space. However, it is only carried out by orthodontists and is not to be carried out by orthodontic therapists.
- *Adjust active components on a removable appliance*:
  - No therapist should be activating active components on a removable appliance. This is only for an orthodontist to do, although after activation they can be inserted by a therapist.
- *Place bends in archwires*:
  - In the final detailing stage of fixed appliance treatment, sometimes bends within a stainless-steel or beta-titanium archwire are needed to help with tooth movement. Any bends are only to be done by an orthodontist; therapists are not allowed to do this.

Any therapist who does not work to their scope of practice and who carries out any procedures from the list of what therapists cannot do is not working in the patient's best interest and will therefore be seen as unfit to practice by the GDC, resulting in them being struck off the register, sued, and possibly no long being able to work in the profession.

50.7 Equality and Diversity

In 2010 the Equality Act replaced the Race Relations Act 1976 and the Disability Discrimination Act 1995 and made them into one Act. The Equality Act aims to strengthen the law by ensuring that every workplace has a fair environment with which all employers and employees comply. There are nine protected characteristics to prevent different forms of discrimination.

50.7.1 Nine Protected Characteristics

The Act protects people from discrimination on the basis of 'protected characteristics':
- *Age*:
  - The Act protects employees of all ages, although this is the only protected characteristic that will allow employers to justify direct discrimination.
- *Disability*:
  - The Act protects anyone who may have a disability to ensure they are treated equally and fairly.
- *Gender*:
  - Anyone who starts or completes the process of a sex change should be treated equally and fairly without any discrimination in their duties at work.
- *Marriage and civil partnership*:
  - The Act protects employees who are married or in a civil partnership against discrimination. Single people are not protected.
- *Pregnancy and maternity*:
  - The Act protects women who are pregnant or who have given birth against discrimination.
- *Race*:
  - The Act protects employees against discrimination based on their race, such as their colour, nationality, or ethnic or national origin.
- *Religion or belief*:
  - The Act protects employees against any discrimination based on their religion or beliefs.
- *Sex*:
  - The Act protects both men and women from any discrimination or paying them differently for the same job just because of their sex.
- *Sexual orientation*:
  - The Act protects bisexual, gay, heterosexual, and lesbian people from any discrimination based on their sexual orientation.

50.7.2 Types of Discrimination

There are six types of discrimination:
- *Direct discrimination*:
  - A person who is treated less favourably than another person because of a protected characteristic.
- *Associative discrimination*:
  - A person who is directly discriminated against because they are associated with someone who has a protected characteristic.
- *Discrimination by perception*:
  - A person who is discriminated against because other people think they have one of the protected characteristics.

- *Indirect discrimination*:
  - When a person is discriminated against by a rule or policy that applies to everyone except them because they have a protected characteristic.
- *Harassment*:
  - When a person suffers offensive behaviour; anyone can complain about behaviour they find offensive, even if it is not directly aimed at them.
- *Victimisation*:
  - When a person has been treated badly and has had to make a complaint or grievance under the legislation.

50.7.3   Strategic Objectives for Equality, Diversity, and Inclusion

The six strategic objectives for all dental professionals within the dental practice are:

- Protect patients through effective regulation.
- Regulate the dental team fairly.
- Be a fair and enabling employer, providing an inclusive and supportive environment for all staff.
- Establish a robust equality and diversity evidence base to inform strategy, policy, and operations.
- Engage the public and stakeholders in the design and delivery of policies and procedures.
- Integrate equality and diversity with governance and management processes.

51

Sharps Injury

Sharps injuries, where a needle, blade, or other sharp object penetrates the skin, can occur in orthodontic practices and it is important that all dental care professionals (DCPs) know what infections can arise and the measures they have to take if there were to be a sharps injury.

The three viral infections of concern following a sharps injury are:

- Human immunodeficiency virus (HIV)
- Hepatitis B
- Hepatitis C.

51.1 Measures to Take Following a Sharps Injury

DCPs who have a sharp injury where the skin has been cut or penetrated by a sharp object that has been in contact with the patient's blood or saliva should take the following first aid measures immediately:

- Stop treatment and encourage bleeding.
- Wash the wound with soap and water, then dry it and cover it with a waterproof dressing.

Once the first two stages have been done, the next actions that should be taken in the management of the sharps injury are:

- Identify the cause.
- Check the patient's medical history and inform the patient if an issue is identified.
- Report the incident to the senior dentist/senior member of staff.
- Telephone the nearest Accident and Emergency, Occupational Health, or Microbiology Department immediately if the patient is a known or suspected carrier of HIV or Hepatitis C for advice and counselling.
- Complete the accident book.

Textbook for Orthodontic Therapists, First Edition. Ceri Davies.
© 2020 John Wiley & Sons Ltd. Published 2020 by John Wiley & Sons Ltd.

51.2   Investigation of Donor and Recipient

Following a sharps injury, both the donor (the patient) and the recipient (the clinician) should be investigated by obtaining the following:

1) 10 ml of clotted blood from the donor, with consent to screen it for blood-borne viruses.
2) 10 ml of clotted blood from the recipient, to be stored for two years.

Counselling should be given to the recipient if necessary.

52

Health and Safety

The Health and Safety at Work Act 1974 lays down the legal framework for health and safety in the UK. The Act stipulates a wide range of duties on employers to protect the health, safety, and welfare of their employees at work. As well as protecting employees, employers also have the responsibility of ensuring that other people on their premises are protected. This includes visitors, temporary workers, casual workers, self-employed workers, clients, and the general public.

The following terms are important in this context:

- *Health* is the protection of bodies and minds from illness resulting from materials, processes, and procedures.
- *Safety* is the protection of people from physical injury.
- *Hazard* is the potential to cause harm.
- *Risk* is the likelihood of causing harm.

52.1 Employer's Duty

Employers have a duty of care to do the following:

- Provide a safe place to work.
- Provide safe equipment.
- Provide safe systems of work.
- Provide safe and competent fellow employees.
- Monitor staff compliance.

52.2 Employee's Duty

Responsibility does not only lie with the employer, it is also the employee's responsibility to take care of themselves by doing the following:

- Use equipment according to instructions.
- Report any imminent danger.
- Report any shortcomings in health and safety.
- Act reasonably to protect their own safety and the safety of others.

52.3 Policies Within the Dental Practice

To ensure health and safety in the dental practice, the following policies must be drawn up:

- Health and safety
- Fire protocol
- Dress code
- Medical emergencies
- Cross-infection control
- Sterilisation procedures
- Immunisation
- Equal opportunities
- Whistle blowing

52.4 Clinical Environment

In the clinical environment there must also be specific health and safety procedures for:

- Clinical waste disposal
- Limiting cross-infection
- Sterilisation procedures
- Personal protective equipment (PPE)
- Risk assessment.

53

Control of Substances Hazardous to Health (COSHH)

The Control of Substances Hazardous to Health (COSHH) Regulations 2002 set out requirements that employers have to abide by to ensure protection of their employees and other people. This includes protection from hazards relating to substances used at work by means of risk assessment, control of exposure, health surveillance, and incident planning. Employees also have the duty to protect themselves and take care of their own exposure to hazardous substances.

Following COSHH guidance is a legal requirement. All employers must have written risk assessments that identify all substances and chemicals, listing:

- The substance.
- Who may be harmed.
- How they may be harmed.
- The level of risk.
- The controls in place.

All staff are required to read and sign the assessment and it must be updated regularly.

54

Reporting of Injuries, Diseases and Dangerous Occurrences (RIDDOR)

The Reporting of Injuries, Diseases and Dangerous Occurrences (RIDDOR) Regulations 2013 require all employers, the self-employed, and others who take responsibility for premises to report any of a range of specified workplace incidents.

All major incidents and dangerous occurrences must be reported to the Health and Safety Executive. Occurrences that must be reported if they arise out of or in connection with work include:

- Death.
- Certain types of injury that result in an employee or self-employed person being absent from work or unable to perform their usual duties.
- Accidents to a person who is not at work, such as patients or visitors.
- Employees or self-employed workers who have an occupational disease.
- Dangerous occurrences which may result in a reportable injury.

55

Consent

Consent is a process in which the patient is enabled to give permission for treatment to be carried out.

55.1 Types of Consent

There are three types of consent:

- *Implied consent*: where, by their actions, a patient appears to agree to a procedure.
  - A scenario for this would be where the patient turns up to the appointment and sits in the dental chair.
- *Expressed consent*: where, by following direct questioning, a patient agrees to a procedure.
  - A scenario for this would be where the procedure for the appointment is given verbally to the patient and they verbally consent to having the treatment done.
- *Informed consent*: where a patient is provided with sufficient and reliable information, in a way they can understand, to be able to make the best decision for their individual needs.
  - A scenario for this is where the patient has been informed of all the risks and benefits, aims, and limitations of orthodontic treatment and consents to the proposed treatment that is in their best interest.

These types of consent are now explained in more detail.

55.1.1 Implied Consent

55.1.1.1 When?

- Consent is gained at every stage of treatment, from referral to discharge.
- Implied consent is gained from the patient at the first visit (assessment) and at the beginning of every appointment.
- No procedures can be done on the basis of implied consent.

55.1.1.2 How?

- The patient turning up to the appointment and sitting in the chair gives implied consent – this shows that the patient has some understanding of why they are there.
- Implied consent is also gained at the beginning of every appointment by the patient showing up and sitting in the chair.

Textbook for Orthodontic Therapists, First Edition. Ceri Davies.
© 2020 John Wiley & Sons Ltd. Published 2020 by John Wiley & Sons Ltd.

- The patient is consenting by their action of turning up to the appointment.
- Implied consent is gained voluntarily: the patient has willingly turned up and has shown that they have some knowledge of where they are and why they are there.

55.1.2 Expressed Consent

55.1.2.1 When?

- At every stage of treatment, from referral to discharge.
- Expressed consent must be gained at the patient's first visit for the clinical examination.
- Expressed consent must be gained at every stage of treatment if there are no changes to the planned treatment.
- All treatment stages are identified to the patient and the information given to obtain consent revisited to assist the patient with their ongoing consent.

55.1.2.2 How?

- Expressed consent is gained verbally and is documented on the patient's clinical records.
- It provides a better safeguard for the dental professional and the patient than implied consent alone.
- Expressed consent is obtained at the first visit for the clinical examination and at every stage of treatment (appointments) for procedures taking place:
  - Explaining the reasons for the examination and the procedures needed at every appointment stage helps the patient understand what is happening.
  - To give consent the patient must express their thoughts and feelings and agree that they are happy to go ahead with the procedure, once they have the ability to understand and voluntarily agree by themselves. This is achieved by engaging them fully in the conversation, which helps to check their understanding by answering any questions they have and asking questions to show their ability to understand.

55.1.3 Informed Consent

55.1.3.1 When?

- Informed consent must be gained at the first visit on the patient journey, the clinical examination. Informed consent must be gained for radiographic examination, impressions, and photographs.
- Informed consent is gained prior to commencing treatment.
- Informed consent is needed again during the stages of treatment if there are any changes to the patient's treatment plan.
- All treatment stages must be identifiable to the patient and revisiting the information given to obtain consent will help assist the patient with their ongoing consent.

55.1.3.2 How?

- Informed consent can be gained verbally or in writing:
  - *Verbal*: by engaging the patient in conversation to check their understanding, by answering questions and asking questions, all of which is documented on the clinical records.
  - *Written*: information in writing signed by the patient or guardian and the clinician, which is required for best practice.

- The risks and benefits, aims and limitations, length, and cost of the treatment, the patient's commitment and compliance, and the option to have no treatment must be explained in terms and language appropriate to the patient's level of understanding. This is also important as it prepares the patient for what is expected of them.
- For informed consent to be obtained and to be valid, it must be voluntarily expressed by a patient or parent/carer who has the ability to understand the proposed treatment. The patient must receive enough information to make the decision voluntarily themselves and must not be pressurised into it. The use of typodonts, photographs, and study models of previous cases can demonstrate the proposed treatment and contribute to the patient's ability to understand.

55.2 Why Do We Obtain Consent?

We obtain consent for the following reasons:

- Ethical and moral obligations to the patient: it protects the patient and their right to choose.
- Legal requirement: Care Quality Commission (CQC) outcome 2 and regulation 18 of the Health & Social Care Act 2008.
- Helps protect the patient and the dental professionals involved in the patient's treatment.

55.3 When Do We Obtain Consent?

Consent must be obtained at every stage of treatment, right from referral up to the patient being discharged. Prior to referral the dentist may gain consent to sharing the patient's information. Patients can withdraw consent at any time; if they do, clinicians must respect this choice.

- First visit (assessment):
  - Implied consent – patient has turned up to appointment.
  - Expressed consent – clinical examination.
  - Informed consent – radiographic examination and impressions. Consent is both verbal and documented in clinical records.
- Prior to commencing treatment:
  - Informed consent – verbal and documented in the clinical records.
  - Written consent form signed by both parent/carer of patient, patient, and clinician; backs up best practice.
- At every stage of treatment:
  - Expressed consent – if no changes to planned treatment; verbal and documented in clinical records.
  - Informed consent – if any changes to treatment plan, new verbal and documented consent is required; best practice is for this to be backed up with a written consent form signed by patient/parent or carer and clinician.
  - Important that all treatment stages are identifiable to patient and that revisiting the information given to obtain consent is used to assist patients with their ongoing consent.

55.4 Who Can Give Consent?

- If the patient is under the age of 16 years, they must either demonstrate Fraser competency in order to consent themselves, or if not their parent/guardian must consent on their behalf.

- Fraser competency is a process by which the clinician can demonstrate that a patient has understood the risks and benefits, aims, and limitations of the proposed treatment to such a degree that they can make the best decision for themselves.
- Patients over the age of 16 years can legally consent to treatment, but it is the clinician's duty of care to make sure they have fully understood the risks and benefits, aims, and limitations of the proposed treatment.
- For patients over the age of 18 years whose ability to understand the proposed treatment is compromised due to learning difficulties, the clinician should assess this and reach a decision about what is in the patient's best interests. No adult can consent on behalf of another adult.
- All members of staff should be involved in the consent process.

55.5 How Can Consent Be Obtained?

There are two types of methods to gain consent:

- *Verbal*: where the patient verbally expresses consent to go ahead.
- *Written*: where the patient, parent or guardian, and clinician sign a written consent form for treatment. This represents best practice.
- In order for consent to be valid, it must be voluntarily expressed:
  - Patients must never be pressured into orthodontic treatment.
  - They must make their own decision.
  - To achieve valid consent the patient or parent/guardian must have the ability to understand the proposed treatment.

All of this equals *valid consent*.

56

Pain and Anxiety Control

Pain and anxiety control can play a big part in orthodontics. It is important that the patient is aware that orthodontic treatment is not always pain free and that some patients can experience discomfort and tenderness from the teeth moving. Anxiety can be a factor in treatment too, so it is important to ensure that the patient is cooperative, since if not treatment can become difficult and the length of treatment may be longer.

To provide some definitions:

- *Pain* is a highly unpleasant physical sensation caused by illness or injury, or it can be mental suffering or distress.
- *Anxiety* is a feeling of worry, nervousness, or unease about something with an uncertain outcome, or a strong desire or concern to do something or for something to happen.

Orthodontic therapists must make sure that each patient is treated the same and that they are all made aware of what to expect with orthodontic treatment. Some patients may come across as very nervous and/or anxious. If this is the case, therapists should ensure that they reassure their patients by explaining every detail of what to expect throughout the appointment, after each appointment, and throughout the rest of the treatment. Because some people are very nervous about dental treatment, some patients are sedated when they undergo treatment, although this is not used in a specialist orthodontic practice. The only place that this may be a possibility is in hospitals for patients who struggle with anxiety, or those with mental or physical disabilities.

56.1 Pain Control

It is important to explain to the patient when they may feel a little pain and how to control it.

Pain may be felt at any stage of treatment, for example:

- *Fitting separators*: pressure may be felt as the separators are being placed between the contact points.
- *Bond-up appointment*: tenderness may be experienced by the evening after the appointment and can last for anything up to a week.
- *Archwire changes*: pressure may be felt from tying the archwire in and the area may be tender by the evening after the appointment, lasting for a couple of days.

Textbook for Orthodontic Therapists, First Edition. Ceri Davies.
© 2020 John Wiley & Sons Ltd. Published 2020 by John Wiley & Sons Ltd.

The patient may want to take medication to help with pain relief, such as:

- Paracetamol/Calpol
- Nurofen
- Ibuprofen – this will also settle any inflammation
- Aspirin (over age of 16).

It is important to ensure that patients who may be allergic to some of these medications do not take them. When discussing this with the patient, check their medical history and advise them that they can use what they usually take at home for pain relief. Asthmatics should not take any ibuprofen.

56.2 Anxiety Control

Some patients suffer from anxiety and this can cause difficulty in orthodontic treatment. Patients have orthodontic treatment because they want it, not because they need it. Those who really want the treatment cooperate better than those who are not too worried if they have treatment or not. Patient cooperation must be at a high level. If you find there is poor cooperation, then consider delaying treatment.

56.2.1 Role of the Orthodontic Therapist in Anxiety Control

Patients may be apprehensive during the early stages of treatment, as they do not know what to expect. Orthodontic therapists must explain what they are going to do to make sure the patient feels reassured. Each patient should have every procedure explained to them in terms of what is going to happen, what will they feel, and so on. For example:

- *Fitting separators*: pressure will be felt as the separators are placed between the contact points, like there is food caught between the teeth.
- *Fitting bands*: pressure will be felt during the placement of bands, which is just ensuring that the bands are fitting flush around the tooth.
- *Taste of glue*: it is important that the patient tries to keep their tongue still, as the materials used do not taste very nice and if glue gets on the tongue the patient will taste it.
- *Impressions*: explain to the patient that the impression will make the mouth feel full.

56.2.2 Bond-up Appointment

At this appointment it is again important to explain each stage and what the patient will feel:

- Preparing teeth:
  - *Cheek retractor*: explain that this will pull on the lips, moving them out the way so the orthodontist can have a better view of the teeth. Reassure the patient that once in place it will feel more comfortable.
  - *Pumice and handpiece*: explain that it is just toothpaste and a toothbrush and it will only be cleaning the teeth like they would be doing at home.
  - *Etch*: explain what it is; some etch comes in the form of what looks like a needle, so reassure the patient that it is not a needle and show them how it works before it is used.
  - *Three in one*: advise it is only air and water; show the patient what it does before it is used.
  - *Suction*: explain to the patient it is like a vacuum cleaner; show them prior to use by testing it on their hand so they know what it is.

- *Fitting brackets*: explain what it feels like when putting them on, how they stick to the teeth, and that a special light makes them stick.
- *Tying in archwire*: explain that the patient may feel a little pressure while the archwire is being engaged into the bracket slots.
- *Instructions*: explain all instructions, reassure the patient that they will be fine, with possible discomfort for a few days or anything up to a week, and that the teeth may be tender.

56.2.3   Adjustment Appointments

At these appointments it is important to do the following:

- Be confident – a confident therapist will allow the patient to feel more reassured and relaxed during appointments.
- Ask the patient how they are, and how they have been getting on.
- Explain to the patient that today will be quick and easy and not as long as the first appointment.
- Recap how well they did at their bond-up appointment.
- Explain what you are going to do today, for example: 'Do you remember when I put your archwire in? That is all we are going to be doing today, but changing to a different wire.'
- Tell the patient what they going to feel, explain that pressure may be felt from tying in the archwire, and that the area may be tender for a couple of days after, but will settle down.
- After the first appointment the patient will be used to seeing you and will know what to expect at appointments, so they will be less anxious.

57

Emergency Care

At some point during orthodontic treatment, a patient may experience an emergency. At all times patients should be careful with their brace, but it is important to ensure that patients are not having regular breakages as this can delay treatment time.

When seeing a patient for an emergency appointment, the following procedure should be carried out:

- Check patient's medical history.
- Make sure the patient knows who you are.
- Find out what the problem is.
- Assess the state of the appliance and the problem.
- Keep things simple and aim to get the patient comfortable.

Note that medical emergencies are addressed in Chapter 59.

57.1 Clinical Problems

57.1.1 Removable Appliances

- *Mouth watering:*
  - Reassure the patient that the more they wear the appliance, the easier it will become. Mouth watering will improve as they get used to the appliance being in the mouth.
- *Speech unclear (patient may lisp):*
  - Reassure the patient that the more they wear the appliance, the more their speech will improve as they get used to the appliance being in the mouth,
- *Appliance loose:*
  - Adjusting the clasps (usually Adams clasps) of a loose-fitting appliance will help with the seating of the appliance in the mouth and make the fit more snug for the patient.
- *Metal component digging into the gum:*
  - Adjusting the clasp and bending it back will prevent it from fitting tightly and digging into the side of the patient's gum.
- *Metal component fractured:*
  - First, assess how fractured the component is. Does it need repairing?
  - If so, an impression will need to be taken for the repair and sent off to the lab with the appliance.

Textbook for Orthodontic Therapists, First Edition. Ceri Davies.
© 2020 John Wiley & Sons Ltd. Published 2020 by John Wiley & Sons Ltd.

– The disadvantage of this is that the patient will have nothing to wear up until the appliance has been repaired, resulting in possible relapse.
- *Acrylic fracture:*
  – First assess how fractured the acrylic is. Does it need repairing?
  – If so, an impression will need to be taken for the repair to be sent off to the lab with the removable appliance.
  – The disadvantage of this is that the patient will have nothing to wear until the appliance has been repaired, resulting in possible relapse.
- *Roof of mouth sore:*
  – The patient may not be cleaning the palate surface area of the appliance properly, so the extent of cleaning needs to be assessed.
  – Advise the patient to clean the palate surface of the removable appliance to prevent soreness and irritation on the mucosa.

57.1.2 Functional Appliances

Functional appliances face similar difficulties to removable appliances, with additional problems including:

- *Teeth/jaw aching:*
  – Reassure patient that they are experiencing this due to the appliance working in the appropriate way, that this is normal, and that the more they wear the appliance, the more they will get used to it and it will settle down. Advise them to take paracetamol, Nurofen, or ibuprofen for the pain.
- *Appliance comes out during the day:*
  – The appliance may be too loose; consider tightening the clasps so the appliance fits snugly in the mouth.
  – Advise full-time wear, as otherwise the appliance will not achieve the desired results.
- *Appliance comes out during the night:*
  – The patient may not be wearing it during the day, so it comes out or they may be removing it during the night in their sleep.
  – Advise full-time wear and check the fit of the appliance, to ensure it is not too loose.
- *Brace digging in:*
  – If the clasp is digging into the patient's gum, bend it down to prevent this, as the appliance may be too tight.
  – If the acrylic is digging into the patient's gum, adjust it with acrylic bur and handpiece and smooth down the acrylic so it does not rub.

57.1.3 Fixed Appliances

57.1.3.1 Wires

- *Long wire (wire sticking out of back bracket):*
  – Cut down the end of archwire at the distal end to make it comfortable for the patient, or singe the back ends of the archwire with a hammer head.
- *Teeth have moved due to wire becoming unengaged from the bracket:*
  – Re-engage the archwire to the bracket slot to help realign the tooth/teeth.
  – Drop down an archwire size to a more flexible archwire to help realign the tooth/teeth.

- *Wire has shifted round to one side:*
  - Remove the archwire and reinsert.
  - Bend the archwire ends with a hammer head.
  - Squeeze crimpable stops to prevent the archwire from sliding from side to side.
- *End of ligature tie turned out:*
  - Turn in the end of ligature ties under the archwire so it does not feel sharp on the patient's tongue.
- *Ligature/module comes off/is loose:*
  - Replace the ligature/module.
  - Using a figure of 8 module increases the friction.
  - Modules cause more friction than stainless-steel ligatures.

57.1.3.2 Bands

- *Bands become loose or fractured:*
  - Rebond the band back or replace with a new one if lost.
  - Replace a fractured band with a new band.
- *Bracket loose/lost:*
  - Rebond the bracket back on or leave until the next visit and cut the wire distal to the bracket mesial to the bracket that has come off.

57.1.3.3 Allergies

- *Patient attends with swollen cheeks*:
  - Check with the orthodontist and refer the patient for a possible allergic reaction.
  - The orthodontist will probably want to debond the patient's appliance.

57.1.3.4 Nance, Quadhelix, and Transpalatal Arch

- Fractured appliance:
  - Remove and smooth down any sharp ends with acrylic bur or by the use of composite on the sharp area.
- *Appliance embedded in the palate* (Figure 57.1):
  - Ask the orthodontist to remove the appliance or refer to them to remove it if they are not on the premises. Orthodontic therapists are not allowed to do this.
  - If there is no orthodontist present, refer the patient to the Accident and Emergency Department or to their general dentist.
- *Appliance dislodged from palatal sheath.*
- *Appliance has become loose:*
  - Clean appliance and rebond.

57.1.3.5 Teeth

- *Teeth feel loose/mobile:*
  - Reassure patient this is normal and that there is always some mobility within the teeth during orthodontics, as the treatment is moving teeth and constantly remodelling the alveolar bone around them. Once the braces are off all the bone hardens up around the teeth.
  - Refer to the orthodontist to check for root resorption.

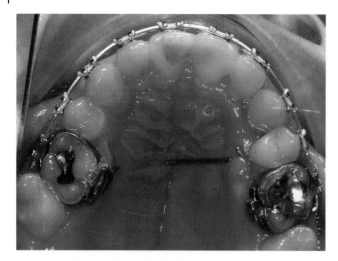

Figure 57.1 Embedded transpalatal arch.

- *Teeth feel loose/painful:*
  - Reassure the patient this is normal and that when teeth are being moved they can become painful/sensitive, especially at the start of treatment.
  - Advise the use of sensitive toothpaste and paracetamol, Nurofen, and ibuprofen for the pain if necessary.
  - Refer to the orthodontist to check and possibly to prescribe an X-ray to check for root resorption.
- *Displaced teeth due to a fall/knock:*
  - Refer to orthodontist, who may suggest placing a flexible wire (0.014/0.016 in. copper nickel titanium) to realign the tooth/teeth.
  - The orthodontist may want to prescribe an X-ray to check if any damage has occurred to the tooth.
  - Tooth vitality must be reviewed and checked if a tooth has had a knock.
  - No heavy forces are to be placed on the tooth/teeth for at least three months if vulnerable.

57.1.3.6 Trauma

- *Loose brackets/bonded brackets causing ulceration:*
  - Remove loose brackets until the next visit to allow the ulcer to settle down.
  - Advise the use of orthodontic wax, rinsing with warm salty water in the area, or the use of Bonjela, which will help settle down the ulcer.
  - Rubbing from the start of initial treatment is normal, as the mouth is not used to having the brace and will need up to a week to settle down.
- *Long wire causing ulceration:*
  - Cut down the long end of archwire with distal end cutters.
  - Advise the use of orthodontic wax on the area to prevent ulceration.
  - Once the wire has been cut down, advise rinsing with warm salty water or the use of Bonjela, which will help to settle down the ulcer.

57.1.3.7 Headgear

- *Appliance is broken:*
  - Cease wear and refer to the orthodontist.
- *Appliance dislodges during the night:*
  - Cease wear and refer to the orthodontist.

57.1.3.8 Bonded Retainers

- *Retainer has come loose:*
  - Leave it until the next appointment, or remove it if it is sharp or causing a problem for the patient.
  - Repair a bonded retainer.
- *Patient is unable to get on with the retainer:*
  - Refer to the orthodontist, who may suggest removing a bonded retainer if the patient cannot get on with it. Explain the risks of not having a bonded retainer. Advise wearing a removable retainer every single night for 10–12 hours a night, otherwise the teeth will move back.
- *Retainer causing irritation to the tongue:*
  - Reassure the patient that this is normal, it just takes time to get used to the retainer.
  - If the patient really cannot cope with it, remove a bonded retainer, but advise wear of a removable retainer every single night for 10–12 hours a night, otherwise the teeth will move back.

58

Orthodontic Instruments

58.1 Adams Spring-Forming Pliers

- Made from extra-hard stainless steel with tungsten carbide inserts on beaks to prolong life.
- One beak round and other beak rectangular (Figure 58.1).
- Used to form and adjust springs on a removable appliance – active components.
- Sterilised by autoclaving, then placed in instrument lube to prevent rusting.

58.2 Adams Universal Pliers

- Made from extra-hard stainless steel with tungsten carbide inserts on beaks to prolong life.
- Both beaks rectangular (Figure 58.2).
- Used to adjust springs and clasps on removable appliances and facebows on headgear.
- More robust than spring-forming pliers.
- Sterilised by autoclaving, then placed in instrument lube to prevent rusting.

58.3 Weingart Pliers

- Made from stainless steel with hard chrome plating (Figure 58.3).
- Used to insert and remove archwires.
- Also used to turn in/down distal ends of archwires.

58.4 Bird Beak Pliers

- Made of stainless steel with short and fine beaks like a bird's beak (Figure 58.4).
- Used to bend fine archwires for fixed appliances.
- Not for use with removable appliances.

Textbook for Orthodontic Therapists, First Edition. Ceri Davies.
© 2020 John Wiley & Sons Ltd. Published 2020 by John Wiley & Sons Ltd.

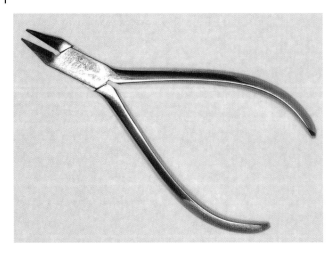

Figure 58.1   Adams spring-forming pliers.

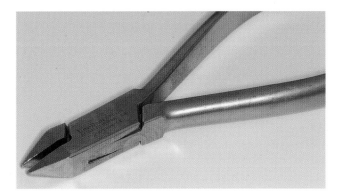

Figure 58.2   Adams universal pliers.

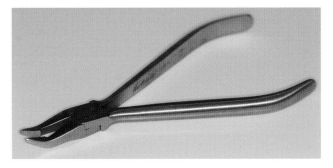

Figure 58.3   Weingart pliers.

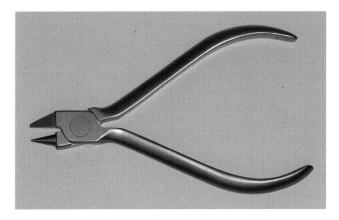

Figure 58.4 Bird beak pliers.

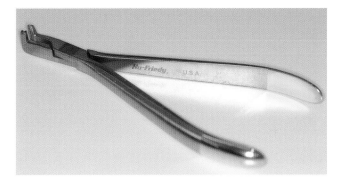

Figure 58.5 Distal end cutters.

58.5 Distal End Cutters

- Made from stainless steel and chrome plated with tungsten carbide inserts (Figure 58.5).
- Used to cut ends of archwire.
- Inserted into mouth at right angle and cut wire distally close to the buccal tube.
- Cut and hold archwire, with inbuilt safety feature preventing inhalation of archwire.

58.6 Ligature Cutter

- Made from stainless steel and hard chrome plating (Figure 58.6).
- Has tungsten carbide inserts.
- Used to cut ligature wires only, never used on archwires.

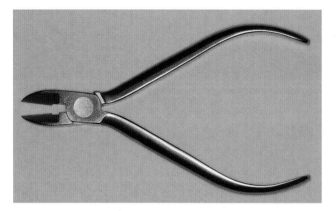

Figure 58.6 Ligature cutter.

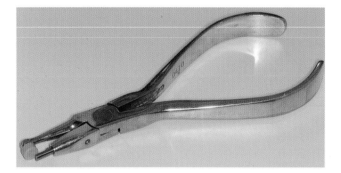

Figure 58.7 Posterior band-removing pliers.

58.7 Posterior Band-Removing Pliers

- Made from stainless steel and hard chrome plating.
- Used to remove molar bands.
- Occlusal stop on pliers placed on occlusal surface of teeth and other arm placed underneath molar band to break free cement and band itself (Figure 58.7).

58.8 Band Pusher

- Also known as a Mershon band pusher.
- Made from stainless steel (Figure 58.8).
- Used to help seat band around tooth.

58.9 Band Seater

- Also known as a bite stick.
- Made from nylon (Figure 58.9).
- Used to help seat molar band around tooth when cementing band.
- Autoclavable.

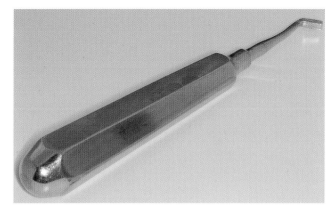

Figure 58.8   Band pusher.

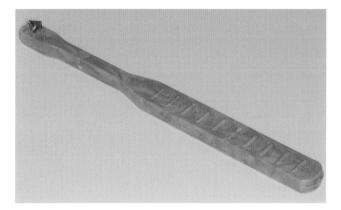

Figure 58.9   Band seater.

58.10   Reverse-Action Bonding Tweezers

- Made from stainless steel (Figure 58.10).
- Hold brackets securely for bonding.
- Squeeze tweezers to open.
- Bracket held in tweezers for loading with adhesive.
- Other end of tweezer tip fits into bracket slot for height adjustment on tooth.

58.11   Torquing Turret

- Stainless-steel hand instrument.
- Used to form arch shape in straight length of wire.
- Can be used to place torque in archform into rectangular archwire.

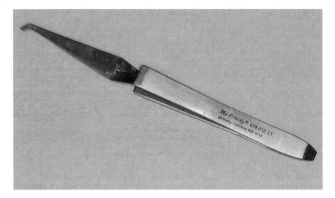

Figure 58.10   Reverse-action bonding tweezers.

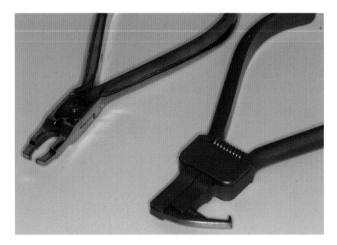

Figure 58.11   Bracket-removing pliers.

58.12   Bracket-Removing Pliers

- Made from extra-hard stainless steel with tungsten carbide inserts on beaks to prolong life (Figure 58.11).
- Used to remove brackets, including lingual brackets.
- Beaks fit around bracket tie wings.

58.13   Nylon Bracket-Removing Pliers

- Made from nylon.
- Fine wire found between beaks – wire replaceable.
- Used to remove brackets – lift off.
- Autoclavable.

58.14   Angled Bracket-Removing Pliers

- Made from stainless steel with hard chrome plating (Figure 58.12).
- Used to remove brackets.
- Beaks placed around bracket tie wings, which help to remove them.

58.15   Dividers

- Made from stainless steel (Figure 58.13).
- Used to measure spaces, arch expansion, or tooth widths, either in mouth or models.

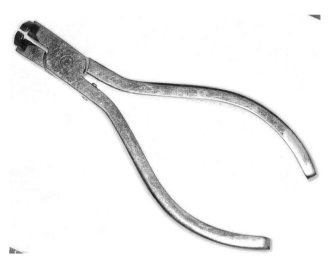

Figure 58.12   Angled bracket-removing pliers.

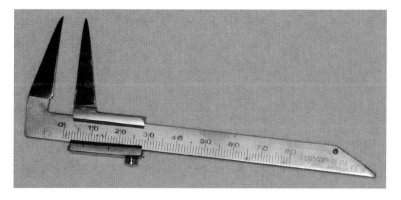

Figure 58.13   Dividers.

58.16   Boon Gauge

- Made from stainless steel.
- Used to measure heights of brackets on each tooth.
- Fine points fixed into each arm at different heights (Figure 58.14).
- Autoclavable.

58.17   Micro Etcher

- Commonly called a sand blaster (Figure 58.15).
- Helps clean and prepare tooth surface or fixed appliances.

58.18   Flat Plastic

- Stainless steel instrument (Figure 58.16).
- Used to load orthodontic bands with cement and apply adhesive to brackets.
- Aid to placement of bonded retainer.

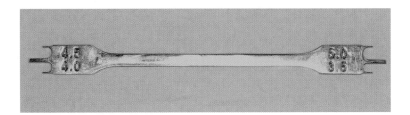

Figure 58.14   Boon gauge.

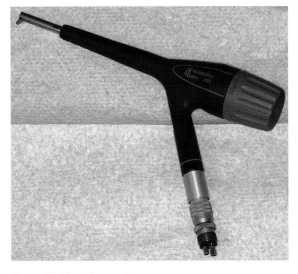

Figure 58.15   Micro etching.

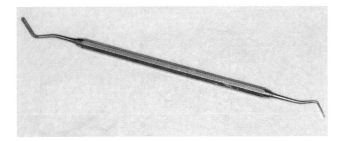

Figure 58.16 Flat plastic.

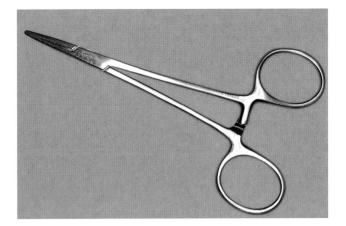

Figure 58.17 Mosquitoes.

58.19 Tweed Loop-Forming Pliers

- Made from stainless steel with hard chrome plating.
- To place loops into rectangular archwires.

58.20 Mosquitoes

- Made from stainless steel with hard chrome plating (Figure 58.17).
- Mainly used for elastic auxiliaries.
- Metal auxiliaries can ruin pliers.
- Can be used for placement of elastomeric modules, placement of separators, and placement of closing nickel titanium retraction springs.

58.21 Mathieu Needle Holders

- Made from stainless steel with hard chrome plating (Figure 58.18).
- Used to hold 'quick ligs' or long ligatures to place them on brackets.
- Use for metal auxiliaries only.

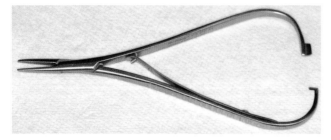

Figure 58.18   Mathieu needle holders.

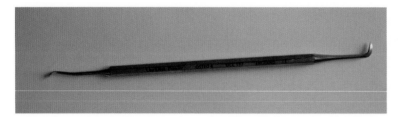

Figure 58.19   Mitchell's trimmer.

58.22   Mauns Heavy-Duty Wire Cutters

- Made from stainless steel.
- Rust very easily.
- To cut any wire size.
- Not to be used inside mouth.

58.23   Mitchell's Trimmer

- Used to remove excess cement from teeth once bands have been cemented (Figure 58.19).
- Used for removal of composite and cement at debonding.

58.24   Separating Pliers

- Also known as coon-style pliers.
- Stainless steel with hard chrome plating (Figure 58.20).
- To place separators between teeth to create space for bands.

58.25   Cheek Retractors

- Made of clear plastic (Figure 58.21).
- Used to retract lips and cheeks during bond-up.
- Cold sterilised can be autoclaved, but doing so tends to make them brittle and they snap.

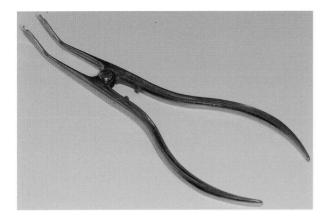

Figure 58.20 Separating pliers.

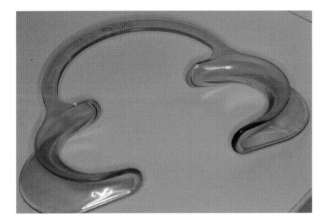

Figure 58.21 Cheek retractors.

58.26 Stainless-Steel Ruler

- Used to measure overjet and overbite in mouth and on models (Figure 58.22).

58.27 Triple-Beak Pliers

- Stainless steel with hard chrome plating (Figures 58.23 and 58.24).
- Used to place small kink into archwire.
- Used for adjustments to quadhelix in mouth.

58.28 Tweeds Straight (Torquing) Pliers

- Made from stainless steel with hard chrome plating (Figure 58.25).
- Used to add small bends in rectangular archwire and for applying torque to archwire by using two pliers together on opposite sides of wire.

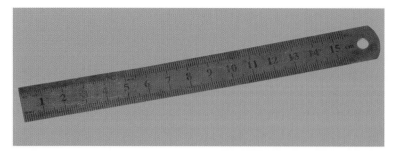

Figure 58.22 Stainless-steel ruler.

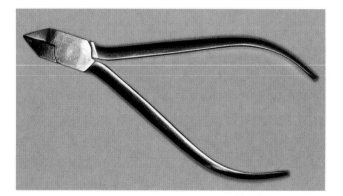

Figure 58.23 Triple-beak pliers.

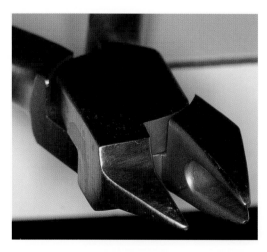

Figure 58.24 Triple-beak pliers.

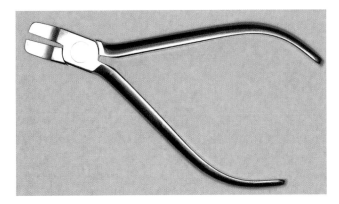

Figure 58.25 Tweeds straight (torquing) plier.

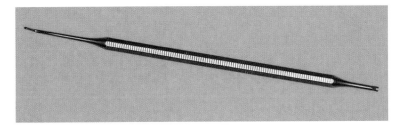

Figure 58.26 Tucker.

- Buccal root torque – archwire twisted forward.
- Palatal root torque – archwire twisted backward.

58.29 Tucker

- Made from stainless steel (Figure 58.26).
- Directs and tucks ends of ligature archwires.

58.30 Photographic Cheek Retractors

- Made from plastic (Figure 58.27).
- Used in pairs to hold cheeks and lips out of way while taking photographs.
- Autoclavable, but can become brittle with time.
- Cold sterilise.

58.31 Photo Mirrors

- Shaped mirrors (Figure 58.28).
- Must be handled with care to avoid scratching.
- Used for intra-oral photographs to give full view of arches.
- Autoclavable.

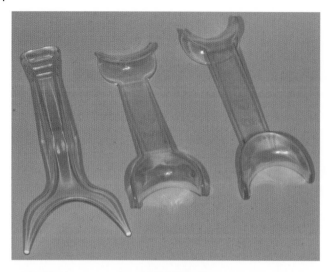

Figure 58.27 Photographic cheek retractors.

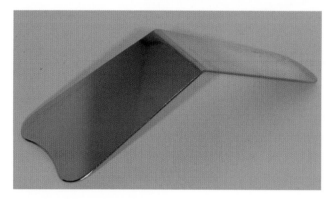

Figure 58.28 Photo mirrors.

58.32 Slow Handpiece

- Made from stainless steel with tungsten carbide coating (Figure 58.29).
- Runs at low speeds and vibrates.
- Speed 40 000 rpm.
- Use latch grip burs.
- Contra angled to use in mouth.
- Does not go through enamel.
- May have water spray to keep tooth cool and fibre-optic light.

58.33 Debond Burs

- Rose head tungsten carbide latch grip bur (Figure 58.30).
- Can come in shape of pear, flame, inverted cone, flat fissure (Figure 58.31), tapered, or bud.
- Used to remove excess composites and cements at debonding.

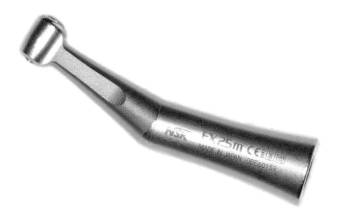

Figure 58.29   Slow handpiece.

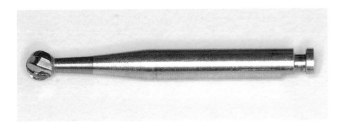

Figure 58.30   Rose head bur.

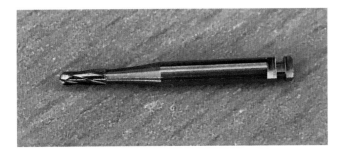

Figure 58.31   Fissure bur.

58.34   Moore's Mandrel

- Made of stainless steel (Figure 58.32).
- Latch grip bur.
- Holds polishing discs.

58.35 Acrylic Bur

- Made from stainless steel (Figure 58.33).
- Friction grip bur.
- Used in straight headpiece.
- Used on acrylic of removable appliance.

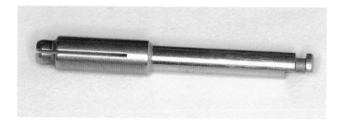

Figure 58.32 Moore's mandrel.

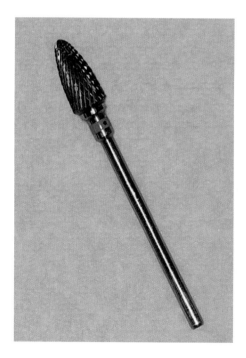

Figure 58.33 Acrylic bur.

59

Medical Emergencies

Medical emergencies can occur at any time, so it is important for every clinician to know what to do. When facing a medical emergency the DRS ABCDE approach is used (Table 59.1).

59.1 Common Medical Emergencies in the Dental Practice

- Anaphylaxis
- Asthma
- Cardiac emergencies – heart attack and angina
- Epileptic seizure
- Hypoglycaemia
- Hyperglycaemia
- Stroke
- Syncope
- Choking

Table 59.2 details the signs, management, and treatment of these emergencies.

59.2 Choking Patients

59.2.1 Adults

1) DRS (Danger, Responsiveness, Shout for Help).
2) Ask patient to cough. If that does not help, go to:
   - Back blows × 5
     - Stand behind patient
     - Slightly tilt forward
     - Hold mandible
     - Deliver hard back blow
     - Check
     - Another back blow, check (up to five times).

Textbook for Orthodontic Therapists, First Edition. Ceri Davies.
© 2020 John Wiley & Sons Ltd. Published 2020 by John Wiley & Sons Ltd.

Table 59.1 DRS ABCDE

D – Danger
- Check for any danger near the patient, such as water, wires, equipment, and relatives

R – Responsiveness
- Check if the patient is responsive:
  - Talk to the patient: 'Hello, can you hear me?'
  - If no response in adults or children, pinch the ear lobe or trapezius to assess whether unconscious
  - If no response in babies, blow hard into the face or pinch the ear lobe

S – Shout for Help
- Shout for help, ask someone to bring the medical emergency kit and defibrillator, and ask someone to be ready to dial 999

A – Airway
- Look inside the mouth and check for any foreign objects blocking the airway
- Is there any swelling?

B – Breathing
- Check for breathing by placing your ear to their mouth and look at their chest
- You want to know:
  - Rate – 12–20 breaths per minute in adults and 20–30 in children
  - Pattern – shallow, deep, or equal?

C – Circulation
- Look at the patient's colour
- Check capillary refill (nail bed): press on nail bed, hold for five seconds, and then release. Count how many seconds the blood takes to refill. It should be below two. If over two seconds the patient will have low blood pressure – do *not* use glyceryl trinitrate (GTN) spray in these patients

D – Disability
- Look at level of consciousness:
  - A – Alert: is the patient alert?
  - V – Verbal: can you talk to them?
  - P – Pain: if they are responsive, ask whether they are in pain
  - U – Unresponsive

E – Exposure
- Check for any injuries
- Any rash, bruising, swelling, or weakness (weakness found in stroke patients)
- Check blood sugars if patient is heading to hypoglycaemia

If that has not worked:
- Abdominal thrusts × 5
  - Stand behind patient
  - Place arms around patient between naval and rib cage
  - Pull in and lift up with both arms still around patient
  - Check
  - Thrust, check (up to five times).
3) If both don't work, call 999 for an ambulance and keep repeating the steps until the ambulance comes.
4) If the patient is unconscious and stops breathing, do DRS ABC and call 999.

Table 59.2 Most common medical emergencies.

Medical emergency	Signs and symptoms	Management	Treatment
Anaphylaxis	• Sudden onset • Swelling – lips, eyes, and tongue • Severe wheezing • Stridor – loud, harsh, high-pitched respiratory sound • Hoarse voice – harsh, raspy, or strained voice • Pale • Clammy/sweating • Flushing and pallor • Rash	DRS ABCDE Call 999 for ambulance	*Adrenalin:* • Epipen – adult or junior • Drawn up: Adults 12+ years = 500 µg (0.5 ml of 1 : 1000) Child 6–12 years = 300 µg (0.3 ml of 1 : 1000) Child less than 6 years = 150 µg (0.15 ml of 1 : 1000) Administered in anterolateral aspect of thigh (top of thigh) *Oxygen:* • 15 l/min
Asthma	• Wheezing • Breathlessness • Can't finish a sentence • Blue looking • A lot of shoulder movement	DRS ABCDE Call 999 for ambulance if no response after 2 puffs of inhaler or if severe and life threatening	*Salbutamol:* • 100 µg/puff • 2–10 puffs = 10 seconds between each one • If no response after two puffs, call 999 • Use spacer if patient unable to do it themselves *Oxygen:* • 15 l/min • 10 mins oxygen – 10 mins puff

(Continued)

Table 59.2 (Continued)

Medical emergency	Signs and symptoms	Management	Treatment
Cardiac emergencies – heart attack and angina	*Heart attack:* • Severe crushing central chest pain that may radiate to neck, shoulder, left arm, and back • Pallor and sweating • Nausea/vomiting • Breathlessness *Angina:* • Pain and discomfort in chest • Pain can feel tight, dull, or heavy • Is this their normal pain?	DRS ABCDE Call 999 for a heart attack or if angina does not get better after medication	*Glyceryl trinitrate (GTN) spray:* • Two sprays under tongue • Only give if capillary pressure under 3 *Aspirin:* • 300 mg orally, crushed or chewed • Do not give if patient has stomach ulcers and if they are already on aspirin and blood-thinning tablets • If patient taking aspirin and knows the dosage, can give equal to 300 mg
Epileptic seizure	• Sudden collapse • Loss of consciousness • Jerking movements • Tongue may be bitten • Frothing of the mouth • Urinating themselves • Confused when they come round	DRS ABCDE Call 999 for ambulance if fit is prolonged by more than 5 mins Patient must go home with someone Do not put anything in patient's mouth Do not strain patient Place in recovery position once seizure stopped If seizure not prolonged could be hypoglycaemia, less than 3 mmol/l can cause a seizure	*Buccal midazolam:* • If prolonged seizure (+5 mins) • Inserted via buccal route • 10+ years = 10 mg • 5–10 years = 7.5 mg • 1–5 years= 5 mg If it does not work, reinsert buccal midazolam via other buccal route

Hypoglycaemia	• Shaking/trembling • Slurred speech • Vagueness • Sweating • Double vision • Confusion • Unconsciousness • Aggressive • Children may seem lethargic	DRS ABCDE Check blood sugars at exposure If patient blood sugar is below 3 mmol/l, then patient has low blood sugar, making them hypoglycaemic. If above 3 mmol/l blood sugars are fine Call 999 for ambulance if patient does not respond	*Conscious and able to swallow:* • 10–20 g glucose such as orange juice, fizzy drink, 4 glucose tablets, or glucose gel *Unconscious and unable to swallow:* • Adult or child 8+ years, glucogen 1 mg intramuscularly (IM) • Child up to 8 years = 0.5 mg IM Administer to upper third of thigh Administer glucogel if cannot do IM, placing in buccal sulcus
Stroke	**F** – Face: mouth or eyelid drooped at smile **A** – Arms: raise both arms and hold for 15 seconds, does one go down? **S** – Speech: unable to speak clearly **T** – Test: test all 3 symptoms	DRS ABCDE Call 999 for ambulance immediately Make sure airway clear and place patient in recovery position Do not give any food or drink	*Oxygen:* 15 l/min
Syncope	• Feels faint • Dizziness • Light-headedness • Collapse • Loss of consciousness • Pallor • Sweating • Slow pulse • Low blood pressure • Nausea/vomiting	DRS ABCDE Lie patient flat and elevate legs Loosen tight clothing If unresponsive, check signs of life	*Oxygen:* 15 l/min

59.2.2 Children

1) DRS.
2) Ask the patient to cough. If that has not helped, go to:
   - Back blows × 5
     - Place patient over your knee or stand for a tall patient
     - Support (hold) mandible
     - Tilt patient down
     - Give a harsh back blow
     - Check, back blow, check (up to five times).

   If back blow does not work:
   - Abdominal thrusts × 5
     - Stand or kneel down behind patient (depending on height of child)
     - Place arms around patient between naval and rib cage
     - Pull in and lift up with both arms still around patient
     - Check
     - Thrust, check (up to five times).
3) If both don't work, call 999 and keep repeating the steps until the ambulance arrives.
4) If the patient is unconscious and stops breathing, do DRS ABC and call 999.

59.2.3 Babies

1) DRS
2) Ask the patient to cough if they are old enough to understand. If that does not help, go to:
   - Back Blows × 5
     - Place patient over your arm facing downwards
     - Support (hold) mandible
     - Give back blow
     - Check (tilt patient to the side)
     - Repeat if needed up to five times.

   If back blows do not work:
   - Chest thrusts × 5
     - Lay baby flat on your arm
     - Hard push in and up with two fingers on chest
     - Check (tilt patient to the side)
     - Repeat chest thrusts up to five times.
3) If neither works, call 999 and keep repeating the steps until the ambulance arrives.
4) If the patient is unconscious and stops breathing, do DRS ABC and call 999.
5) With a baby, always get an ambulance to check them after any episode of choking.

If an object is inhaled it will become lodged in the right lung. If this does happen, sit the patient up and encourage them to cough. If the object does not come out, then use back slaps/abdominal thrusts. If the object still has not appeared, then an ambulance needs to be called and oxygen issued. Once the ambulance has arrived, if necessary the patient will be sent to the hospital for further investigation such as a radiograph to locate the object.

59.3 Cardiac Arrest Patients

59.3.1 Adults

DRS ABC:

- *Danger*: check for danger.
- *Responsiveness*: Ask 'Hello, can you hear me?' Pinch ear or trapezius if no response.
- *Shout for help*: ask for medical kit, defibrillator, and ask someone to stand by to phone 999.
- *Airway*: check nothing is obstructing, if not then head tilt and chin lift.
- *Breathing*: pull chin back and up. Put your ear to their mouth to feel their breath and look at their chest. Respiratory rate should be 12–20 bpm.
- *Compressions*: start cardiopulmonary resuscitation (CPR):
  - *Depth*: 5–6 cm.
  - *Rate*: 100–120 per minute.
  - *Ratio*: 30 to 2 breaths.
  - *Position*: Centre of chest, lower third of sternum – hands interlocked.
  - Use the defibrillator and call 999, carry on until an ambulance has arrived.
  - If signs of life occur, then stop CPR, place patient in recovery position, and maintain the airway.

59.3.2 Children

DRS ABC:

- *Danger*: check for danger.
- *Responsiveness*: ask 'Hello, can you hear me?' Look for signs of life, pulse, colour, and any response.
- *Shout for help*: ask for a medical kit, defibrillator, and ask someone to stand by to phone 999.
- *Airway*: check nothing is obstructing, if not then slight extension on head tilt.
- *Breathing*: pull chin back and up. Put your ear to their mouth to feel their breath and look at their chest. Respiratory rate should be 20–30 bpm.
- Compressions: start CPR.
  - *Depth*: 4–5 cm.
  - *Rate*: 120 per minute.
  - *Ratio*: 15 to 2 breaths.
  - *Position*: centre of chest, lower/third of sternum – one hand on child unless a big child, then use two hands.
  - Use defibrillator and call 999, carry on until an ambulance has arrived.
  - If signs of life occur, then stop CPR, place in recovery position, and maintain the airway.

59.3.3 Babies up to 1 Year Old

DRS ABC:

- *Danger*: check for danger.
- *Responsiveness*: scoop baby up opposite you, pinch their ear, and blow hard in their face.
- *Shout for help*: ask for medical kit, defibrillator, and ask someone to stand by to phone 999.

- *Airway*: check nothing is obstructing, if not then keep baby's head in natural alignment, one finger on chin and head level up.
- *Breathing*: lay baby flat and cover their nose and mouth to see if they are breathing.
- *Compressions*: start CPR.
  - *Depth*: 4–5 cm.
  - *Rate*: 120 per minute.
  - *Ratio*: 15 to 2 breaths.
  - *Position*: between the nipple line, two fingers only, tilt head back ever so slightly, not all the way.
  - Call 999 and carry on until an ambulance has arrived.
  - If signs of life occur, then stop CPR, place baby in the recovery position, and maintain the airway.

59.3.4 Pregnant Women

DRS ABC:

- *Danger*: check for danger.
- *Responsiveness*: ask 'Hello, can you hear me?' Pinch ear or trapezius if no response.
- *Shout for help*: ask for medical kit, defibrillator, and ask someone to stand by to phone 999.
- *Airway*: check nothing is obstructing, if not then head tilt and chin lift.
- *Breathing*: pull chin back and up. Put your ear to their mouth to feel their breath and look at their chest. Respiratory rate should be 12–20 bpm.
- *Compressions*: start CPR.
  - *Depth*: 5–6 cm.
  - *Rate*: 100–120 per minute.
  - *Ratio*: 30 to 2 breaths.
  - *Position*: centre of chest, lower third of sternum, hands interlocked. Put patient in the left lateral position at 30°, which takes pressure off the vena cava of the heart and drops the uterus down.
  - Use the defibrillator and call 999, carry on until an ambulance has arrived.
  - If signs of life occur, then stop CPR, place the patient in the recovery position, and maintain the airway.

60

Eruption Dates

All teeth, both deciduous (Table 60.1) and permanent (Table 60.2), have different dates by which they should calcify and by which they should normally erupt.

Root formation for deciduous teeth is usually complete by around 12–18 months, and for permanent teeth by around 24–36 months.

60.1 Deciduous Teeth

Table 60.1 Eruption and calcification dates for deciduous teeth.

Teeth	Eruption	Calcification
A	6 months	
B	7 months	
C	18 months	0–16 weeks in utero
D	12 months	
E	24 months	

Textbook for Orthodontic Therapists, First Edition. Ceri Davies.
© 2020 John Wiley & Sons Ltd. Published 2020 by John Wiley & Sons Ltd.

Table 60.2 Eruption and calcification dates for permanent teeth.

Upper			Lower	
teeth	Eruption	Calcification	teeth	Eruption
1	7 years	3–6 months	1	7 years
2	8 years	10–12 months 3–6 months	2	8 years
3	11 years	3–6 months	3	10 years
4	9 years	1–2 years	4	9 years
5	10 years	1–2 years	5	11 years
6	6 years	Birth	6	6 years
7	12+ years	3 years	7	12+ years
8	18+ years	7 years	8	18+ years

61

Extraction Patterns

Treatment planning can incorporate different extraction patterns. The teeth considered for extraction are all dependent on what type of case it is and how much space is required.

61.1   Class I Cases

Mild to moderate crowding (Figure 61.1):

$$\frac{5 \mid 5}{5 \mid 5}$$

Figure 61.1   Class I, mild to moderate crowding extraction pattern.

$$\frac{4 \mid 4}{4 \mid 4}$$

Figure 61.2   Class I, moderate to severe crowding extraction pattern.

$$\frac{4 \mid 4}{ \mid }$$

Figure 61.3   Class II, mild to moderate crowding extraction pattern.

$$\frac{4 \mid 4}{5 \mid 5}$$

Figure 61.4   Class II, moderate to severe crowding extraction pattern 1.

- All second premolars are taken, as not much space is required.
- Finish in a full unit class I molar relationship.
- Balancing and compensating extractions.

Moderate to severe crowding (Figure 61.2):

- All first premolars are taken, as more space is required.
- Finish in a full unit class I molar relationship.
- Balancing and compensating extractions.

61.2   Class II Cases

Mild to moderate crowding with a well-aligned lower arch (Figure 61.3):

- Upper first premolars taken, since to reduce an overjet more space is required anteriorly.
- Finish in a full unit class II molar relationship.
- Balancing extractions.

Moderate to severe crowding in both arches (Figure 61.4):

- Upper first premolars taken, since to reduce an overjet more space is required anteriorly.
- In skeletal II patients the lower posterior segment is brought forward due to a wish not to make them more class II by retracting the lower teeth.

Textbook for Orthodontic Therapists, First Edition. Ceri Davies.
© 2020 John Wiley & Sons Ltd. Published 2020 by John Wiley & Sons Ltd.

```
4 | 4
——————
4 | 4
```

Figure 61.5 Class II, moderate to severe crowding extraction pattern 2.

Alternatively (Figure 61.5):

- Moderate crowding in the lower arch – lower second premolars.
- Severe crowding in the lower arch – lower first premolars.
- Both will finish in a full unit class I molar relationship.
- Balancing and compensating extractions.

61.3 Class III Cases

```
5 | 5
——————
4 | 4
```

Figure 61.6 Class III, extraction pattern 1.

Figure 61.7 Class III, extraction pattern 2.

Figure 61.8 Class III, extraction pattern 3.

In class III cases, due to lower teeth being more prominent anterior teeth are always considered for extraction to help bring the lower teeth posterior. There are three options.

Either 5s and 4s (Figure 61.6):

- More space required anteriorly on the lower arch.
- Finish in a full unit class I molar relationship.
- Balancing and compensating extractions.

Or, rarely, only 4s (Figure 61.7):

- More space required anteriorly on the lower arch.
- Finish in a full unit class I molar relationship.
- Balancing extractions.

Or, even more rarely, 1s (Figure 61.8).

61.4 Balancing and Compensating Extractions

Balancing extractions are teeth extracted either side of the arch, preventing the dental midline from shifting around to one side of the arch. For example, extracting both upper first premolars.

Compensating extractions are teeth extracted in the opposing arch to manage occlusion. For example, extracting UL5 due to poor prognosis and LL5 to compensate.

62

Tooth Fusion and Gemination

Tooth *fusion* is where two individual teeth are fused together. Each tooth has an individual pulp chamber and root canal.

Tooth *gemination* occurs when two teeth develop together and form one tooth. Visibly the crown of this tooth is large and there is only one root with a single root canal.

Figure 62.1 shows what tooth fusion and gemination look like. The root determines the difference between the two. The only way to tell them apart clinically is by using dental panoramic tomography (DPT), which will help to assess and identify how many roots are present.

Tooth fusion and gemination are most commonly seen in the deciduous dentition, although they are also seen in the permanent dentition, with the incisors being affected.

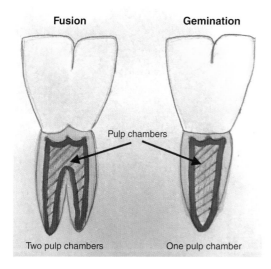

Figure 62.1 Tooth fusion and gemination.

Textbook for Orthodontic Therapists, First Edition. Ceri Davies.
© 2020 John Wiley & Sons Ltd. Published 2020 by John Wiley & Sons Ltd.

62.1 Treatment

Different treatment options are considered for tooth fusion and gemination within the deciduous and permanent dentition.

- Within the deciduous dentition, if the tooth is fused or geminated it may exfoliate itself. However, if it does not, then it should be considered for extraction.
- In the *permanent* dentition, extraction of the fused or geminated tooth is the usual approach in orthodontic treatment.

If the fused or geminated tooth is of a good size and not very wide, then consideration may be given to keeping the tooth. However, it is important to ensure that the dentist advises the patient that they need to maintain good oral hygiene, as there is a risk of the joining of the enamel developing a cavity. Having the crown resized to an acceptable width can be considered, although this is very rarely done.

63

Extra Notes

This chapter contains notes on additional topics that are relevant to orthodontics of which the student may want to be aware.

3D expansion screw	Turn the key one day for the midline and two to three days later for the anterior segment. These are never done at the same time.
Active self-ligating brackets	These give more torque expression in working archwires.
Aesthetic brackets	May be plastic or ceramic. Plastic brackets cannot get any torque expression and they distort.
Annealing nickel titanium archwires	Also known as heating of the archwire until it goes red, which takes all the super-elasticity out of the archwire.
Archwire in class III cases	17 × 25 can be used in class III as torque is not fully expressed in the lower arch.
Assessing archforms	Get pre-treatment models and place archwire on the arch. Use the one with the best fit.
Ball-ended clasps	Used more in functional appliances than Adams clasps due to some molars having no undercuts. Can be used with fixed appliances as they fit under wire.
Bifurcation	Area found under tooth between roots is called the bifurcation area.
Bolton analysis	Looks at tooth size discrepancy and measures widths of canines, laterals, and incisors (3-3). If there is a discrepancy between the upper and lower arches, restorations may be needed.
Bonded retainers	Definitely used in diastemas, rotations, crowding and any high-risk relapse potential cases. Can be made from 0.0175 in. twist-flex wire.
Bonded retainer 2-2	Ideal for class II finish cases, as they knock a bonded retainer off on the canines.
Bonded retainer 3-3	Ideal for class I finish cases.
Bonded retainer 4-4	Used for buccal canines to prevent them from relapsing or when canines are missing.

Textbook for Orthodontic Therapists, First Edition. Ceri Davies.
© 2020 John Wiley & Sons Ltd. Published 2020 by John Wiley & Sons Ltd.

Brown spots	On the teeth, may be caries or lesions.
Cephalometry	Involves taking and analysing a cephalometric radiograph or ceph.
Cinching back archwires	Helps to stop flexible archwires from coming out of the back bracket, but also stops proclination of the anterior segment.
Class III malocclusion	Swapping brackets left and right on canines will help to stop mesial tipping of these teeth. Keep them in round wires on the lower arch to help roll back the lower incisors. Rectangular archwires will procline the lower anterior segment.
Cleft lip and palate	More class III skeletal because the mandible carries on growing, but growth in the maxilla is delayed.
Decalcification	80% of patients have decalcification after orthodontic treatment.
Dental panoramic tomography (DPT)	Panoramic radiograph.
Emergence profile	Correct gingiva will give a good emergence profile, as opposed to a patient who has recession.
Ethyl chloride	Can help to make archwire more flexible for full archwire engagement.
Expansion devices	Removables get more tipping and teeth flare out. With quadhelix and rapid maxillary expander (RME) there is less tipping and teeth move bodily. Widening a rectangular stainless-steel or beta-titanium archwire can achieve expansion, which is useful when correcting crossbites. Headgear is used for expansion of the facebow. X-bite elastics can help widen the upper arch.
Extracting first permanent molars (6s)	These are difficult to extract and shorten the dental arch.
Fluoride	Toothpaste contains 1450 ppm of fluoride.
Fraenectomy	Pull lip up: if the gingival blanches (goes white) palatal to incisors, it means a fraenectomy is needed.
Hawley retainer	Helps with buccal occlusal settling. High-relapse appliance, must be tight against all incisors.
Impacted lower second premolars	Can erupt lingually/palatally.
Implants	7 mm of space is required for an implant.
Informed consent	The following should be within the informed consent: type of appliance, need for retainers, extractions, how often the patient needs to attend, the fact that they need to continue to see their own dentist, risks and benefits, aims and limitations, advantages, disadvantages, alternative treatment, option of no treatment.
Large canines on X-rays	Canines could be palatally placed.
Magnetic resonance imaging (MRI) scans	Braces should be removed for MRI scans as stainless-steel brackets are magnetic. Absolute ceramic brackets are fine.

Mamelons	Found around incisal edges, but get ground down when dentition erupts.
MBT prescription	Wants more torque expression. Bracket slot size 22×28 preferred to 18×25 as can get bowing with thin wires on smaller bracket slot.
Missing upper lateral case	Placing U2 brackets on U3s will place more palatal root torque due to the canine root being more labial. Place canines on premolars to get buccal eminence look. This is considered when camouflaging canines as lateral incisors.
Molar bands	Size of band is always found on its mesial aspect. Use bite stick to seat the band. To check fit is correct, check that band is not rocking and that bracket on band is level with occlusal plane.
Nickel titanium closing springs	Can distort, oral hygiene can be poor. Provide constant force and small degradation in form.
Odontomes	Two types: compound (lots of little clusters) and complex (one large mass).
Offset brackets	Prevent debonding of brackets. Most debonds occur in the premolar region. Bracket base has a bigger surface area.
Picking up second permanent molars (7s)	Doing this will help in a deepbite case (wedge effect).
Pre-adjusted edgewise (prescriptions)	In and out = thicker at base of bracket. Tip = angulation of the bracket slot. Torque (buccolingual) = angulation of the bracket by use of rectangular wires.
Pressure-formed retainers	Cover the occlusal surface, resulting in no occlusal settling. The patient must finish with a good occlusion as no vertical occlusal settling is achieved.
Primary Care Trust (PCT)	For a patient who cannot attend the dental practice, the local PCT should be contacted to see if they could transfer the patient to a local dentist or possibly help with funding. PCTs work with the General Dental Council and deal with staff and government, funding, and complaints.
Problems with camouflaging canines as laterals	They are more yellow in colour, they have a high gingival contour (gingival line), they are wider, and their shape is more bulbous.
Reactivating functionals	There are two ways: chairside, add acrylic to bite blocks; and in the lab, use of new impression and wax bite.
Reducing anterior openbite (AOB): high pull headgear	A wedge effect occurs by intruding the posterior segment in the maxilla, which encourages forward growth rotation of the mandible and a reduction in maxillary-mandibular plane angle (MMPA) and lower anterior facial height (LAFH), with more buccal intrusion reducing the AOB.
Reducing deepbite: low pull headgear	A wedge effect is obtained by extruding the posterior segment in the maxilla, which encourages backward growth rotation of the mandible and an increase in MMPA and LAFH, with more buccal extrusion reducing the deepbite.
Removing a transpalatal arch (TPA)/TPA with Nance	A high-speed handpiece is used to remove interarch wire, and only the orthodontist does this. Leave molar bands on if continuing into fixed appliances.

Self-ligating brackets	An active bracket has an extra metal button on the inside gate which places an active force on the archwire. A passive bracket is where the gate on the bracket is flat and there is no extra metal button, which places no active force on the archwire.
Short roots	Its aetiology could be a disruption of the development of dentition.
Stippled gums	Surface looks like orange peel.
Torque	You can see you have enough torque by palpating the root in the sulcus. If there is not enough a torque bend is to be placed in the archwire.
Transposed teeth	There are two types: false and true transposition. The most commonly transposed teeth are U3s and U4s, and L2s and L3s.
Ways of attaching elastics	Circle loops, U loops, hooks, Kobayashi hooks, posted archwires.

64

Definitions

Molar Relationship

Class I The mesiobuccal cusp of the upper first molar occludes in the buccal groove on the lower first molar.

Class II The mesiobuccal cusp of the upper first molar occludes anterior to the buccal groove of the lower first molar.

Class III The mesiobuccal cusp of the upper first molar occludes posterior to the buccal groove of the lower first molar.

Incisor Relationship

Class I The lower incisor edges occlude with or lie immediately below the cingulum plateau of the upper central incisors.

Class II div I The lower incisor edges occlude posterior to the cingulum plateau of the upper central incisors. The upper central incisors are proclined and there is an increase in the overjet.

Class II div II The lower incisor edges occlude posterior to the cingulum plateau of the upper central incisors. The upper central incisors are retroclined and there is a reduced or increased overjet. The common feature is proclined lateral incisors.

Class III The lower incisor edges occlude anterior to the cingulum plateau of the upper central incisors. The overjet is reduced or reversed.

Canine Relationship

Class I The upper canine occludes and lies in the embrasure between the lower canine and first premolar.

Class II The upper canine occludes anterior and lies in the embrasure between the lower lateral incisors and canine.

Class III The upper canine occludes posterior and lies in the embrasure between the lower first and second premolars.

Textbook for Orthodontic Therapists, First Edition. Ceri Davies.
© 2020 John Wiley & Sons Ltd. Published 2020 by John Wiley & Sons Ltd.

Other Definitions

Hypodontia	Missing teeth, used when there is congenital absence of one or more primary or secondary teeth (missing teeth).
Oligodontia	More than six missing teeth.
Anodontia	Total loss of teeth.
Supernumerary	An extra tooth found when there are excess teeth of the normal series.
Impaction	Failure of eruption of a tooth/canine due to crowding or an obstruction within the dental arch.
Deepbite	Vertical overlap of upper incisors over lower incisors when posterior segment is in occlusion. Upper incisors overlap lower incisors in excess of 4 mm or more.
Normal overbite	Upper incisors cover one-third of lower incisors with posterior segment in occlusion.
Increased overbite	Upper incisors cover more than one-third of lower incisors when posterior segment is in occlusion.
Decreased overbite	Upper incisors cover less than one-third of lower incisors when posterior segment is in occlusion.
Incomplete overbite	Lower incisors do not come into contact with hard or soft tissues.
Complete overbite	Lower incisors do come into contact with hard or soft tissues.
Anterior openbite (AOB)	No vertical overlap of the upper and lower incisors when posterior segment is in occlusion.
Posterior openbite (POB)	No vertical overlap of upper and lower posterior teeth when posterior segment teeth are in occlusion.
Crossbites	An abnormal relationship between opposing teeth in buccopalatal or buccolingual direction.
Posterior crossbite	**B**uccal cusps of lower teeth occlude **b**uccal to **b**uccal cusps of upper teeth when patient is in full occlusion.
Anterior crossbite	One or more of the maxillary incisors occlude lingual to lower incisors with posterior teeth in occlusion.
Lingual crossbite	**B**uccal cusps of lower teeth occlude **p**alatal to **p**alatal cusps of upper teeth when patient in full occlusion.
Overjet	Distance between upper and lower incisors in horizontal plane. Normal overjet is 2–4 mm.

Bimaxillary proclination	Occlusions where both upper and lower incisors are proclined.
Centre of resistance	Point in the body where resistance to movement is concentrated.
Force moment	The component found within a force that causes rotational movement only.
Force couple	In fixed appliances, when an archwire connects into a bracket slot a force couple is created, which will achieve rotation, inclination of teeth, and torque.
Dental panoramic tomography (DPT)	A radiograph that gives a two-dimensional view of the upper and lower jaws (maxilla and mandible).
Cephalometric radiograph	A true lateral view of the skull, a two-dimensional image of a three-dimensional object presenting the skull and facial bones.
Upper standard occlusal radiograph (USO)	A radiograph of the anterior part of the maxilla and anterior teeth.
Parallax	A technique used when assessing or localising the position of unerupted tooth/teeth.
Removable appliance	An orthodontic appliance that can be removed by the patient from the mouth for the maintenance of oral hygiene. Either an active appliance to aid in tooth movement or passive when prescribed as a retainer or as an appliance to maintain space within the arch.
Functional appliance	A fixed or a removable appliance used in class II malocclusions that achieves a forward posture of the mandible, causing stretching of the facial soft tissues to produce a combination of dental and skeletal changes.
Fixed appliance	An orthodontic appliance that is fixed to the teeth and cannot be removed by the patient.
Headgear	An orthodontic appliance that provides extra-oral anchorage and extra-oral traction outside of the mouth via attachment of another orthodontic appliance (fixed or removable).
Anchorage	Control of unwanted tooth movement.
Index of Orthodontic Treatment Need (IOTN)	Used to assess the need for treatment.
Peer Assessment Rating (PAR)	Used to measure the success of treatment.
Cleft lip and palate	A cranio-facial malformation.

Retention   Used to minimise relapse and maintain the result achieved at the end of treatment.

Consent   A process in which the patient is enabled to give permission for treatment to be carried out.

Tooth fusion   Where two individual teeth are fused together. Each tooth has an individual pulp chambers and root canal.

Tooth gemination   When two teeth develop together and form one tooth. Visibly the crown of this tooth is large and there is only one root with a single root canal.

Index

Textbook for Orthodontic Therapists, First Edition. Ceri Davies.
© 2020 John Wiley & Sons Ltd. Published 2020 by John Wiley & Sons Ltd.